TABLE OF CONTENTS

ABBREVIATIONS

ACT	Artemisinin-based combination therapy
AMFm	Affordable Medicines Facility-malaria
ANC	Antenatal care
AL	Artemether-lumefantrine
BCC	Behavior change communication
CCM	Community case management
CDC	Centers for Disease Control and Prevention
CHW	Community health workers
DDSR	Division of Disease Surveillance and Response
DfID	Department for International Development (UK)
DHA-PPQ	Dihydroartemisinin-piperaquine
DHS	Demographic and health survey
DOMC	Division of Malaria Control
DSS	Demographic Surveillance System
FANC	Focused antenatal care
FELTP	Field Epidemiology and Laboratory Training Program
GHI	Global Health Initiative
Global Fund	The Global Fund for HIV/AIDS, Tuberculosis and Malaria
GOK	Government of Kenya
HMIS	Health Management Information System
IDSR	Integrated Disease Surveillance and Response
IEC	Information, education and communication
IPTp	Intermittent preventive treatment for pregnant women
IRS	Indoor residual spraying
ISTp	Intermittent screening and treatment for pregnant women
ITN	Insecticide-treated net
KEMRI	Kenya Medical Research Institute
KEMSA	Kenya Medical Supplies Agency
LMIS	Logistics Management Information System
M&E	Monitoring and Evaluation
MIP	Malaria in pregnancy
MIS	Malaria Indicator Survey
MOP	Malaria Operational Plan
MOPHS	Ministry of Public Health and Sanitation
NMS	National Malaria Strategy
PEPFAR	President's Emergency Plan for AIDS Relief
PMI	President's Malaria Initiative
QA/QC	Quality assurance/quality control
RBM	Roll Back Malaria
RDT	Rapid diagnostic test
SP	Sulfadoxine-pyrimethamine
TWG	Technical Working Group
USAID	United States Agency for International Development
USG	United States Government
WHO	World Health Organization

EXECUTIVE SUMMARY

Malaria prevention and control are major foreign assistance objectives of the U.S. Government (USG). In May 2009, President Barack Obama announced the Global Health Initiative (GHI), a comprehensive effort to reduce the burden of disease and promote healthy communities and families around the world. Through the GHI the USG will improve health outcomes, building upon and expanding the USG's successes in addressing specific diseases and issues.

The President's Malaria Initiative (PMI) is a core component of the GHI, along with HIV/AIDS, maternal and child health, and tuberculosis. PMI was launched in June 2005 as a five-year, $1.2 billion initiative to rapidly scale up malaria prevention and treatment interventions and reduce malaria-related mortality by 50% in 15 high-burden countries in sub-Saharan Africa. With passage of the 2008 Lantos-Hyde Act, funding for PMI has now been extended through FY 2014. Programming of PMI activities follows the core principles of GHI: encouraging country ownership and investing in country-led plans and health systems; increasing impact and efficiency through strategic coordination and programmatic integration; strengthening and leveraging key partnerships, multilateral organizations, and private contributions; implementing a woman- and girl-centered approach; improving monitoring and evaluation; and promoting research and innovation.

A decline in the burden of malaria in Kenya has been observed in recent years resulting in low malaria transmission intensity in most parts of the country. The 2010 Malaria Indicator Survey (MIS) results confirmed that malaria prevalence is nearly three times as high in rural areas (12%) as in urban areas (5%), with documented moderate to high levels of transmission remaining in certain endemic zones. Malaria prevalence in the lake endemic zone remains concerning at 38%, while prevalence in other non-endemic zones has dropped to less than 5%. Consequently, as part of the Division of Malaria Control's (DOMC) 2009-2017 National Malaria Strategy, prevention and control interventions are tailored to the current epidemiology of malaria, with a concentration of efforts in the lake endemic zone.

Kenya submitted a successful application to the Global Fund to Fight AIDS, Tuberculosis and Malaria for a Round 10 malaria grant, which was signed in early 2012 and has a Phase 1 (September 2011-December 2013) value of over $38 million. This new grant will, over the next five years, provide critical support for maintaining universal coverage of insecticide-treated nets, ensuring a nationwide supply of artemisinin-based combination therapy treatments, and rolling out the national diagnostic policy and getting rapid diagnostic tests into lower-level health facilities. The funding does not fully cover commodity and programmatic needs, and the Ministry's Department of Malaria Control (DOMC) will rely on the participation of national and international partners to ensure effective malaria prevention and control in the country. The activities that PMI is proposing for FY 2013 are matched with identified needs and priorities described in the DOMC's National Malaria Strategy (2009-2017) and build on investments designed to improve and expand malaria-related services during the first five years of PMI funding. The proposed FY 2013 PMI budget for Kenya is $32.4 million.

To achieve the goals and targets of the DOMC and PMI, the following major activities will be supported with FY 2013 funding:

Insecticide-treated nets (ITNs): The 2009-2017 National Malaria Strategy promotes universal ITN coverage, defined as one net per two people, within prioritized districts of the country. In 2011, Kenya conducted a rolling mass campaign to scale up to universal coverage of ITNs in priority endemic areas; over 7.6 million ITNs were distributed to priority areas in Nyanza, Western and Rift Valley Provinces, and in 2012 an additional three million will be distributed in Coast Province. Other distribution strategies include free or highly-subsidized ITNs provided through antenatal care (ANC) clinics and the expanded program on immunization services, child health action days, community-based initiatives, and retail outlets. In 2010, household ownership of ITNs was 48%, while proportions of children under five years and pregnant women who slept under an ITN the previous night were 42% and 41% respectively.

By the end of 2012, after five years of implementation, PMI will have purchased a total of over 5.2 million ITNs, of which 1.3 million were purchased in 2012, in support of both Kenya's routine and mass distribution efforts to reach at risk populations. To continue supporting national ITN policies, PMI will procure an estimated 1.3 million ITNs with FY 2013 funding for free routine distribution through ANC clinics and an additional 500,000 for distribution in the 2014 mass campaign. PMI will support the DOMC to continue development of innovative ways to replace worn-out nets at the community level. Additionally, PMI will continue to work with non-governmental organizations on community-based information, education and communication/behavior change communication (IEC/BCC) campaigns to increase demand for ITNs combined with correct and consistent use.

Indoor residual spraying (IRS): PMI has supported the national IRS program since 2007. PMI currently targets four[1] districts in Nyanza Province and protects over 1.2 million people annually. With FY 2013 funding, PMI will continue to support IRS in up to three priority districts in collaboration with the DOMC and the new DfID IRS program. Given the changes occurring in the IRS program, specific program targets will be established in 2013 when more clarity is provided. PMI will support entomological monitoring to detect and respond to resurgences of mosquito populations in districts transitioning away from IRS programs. PMI will also conduct epidemiological surveillance and monitoring in endemic IRS districts at both the facility and community level to enable the DOMC to make informed decisions about its IRS program.

Intermittent preventive treatment of pregnant women (IPTp): The 2010 Malaria Indicator Survey results showed improved though continued low coverage of IPTp—only 25% of pregnant women receive two or more doses of sulfadoxine-pyrimethamine, despite high ANC attendance (86% of women attend ANC two or more times during their pregnancy). In the past year, PMI has trained approximately 2,000 community health workers on focused antenatal care/malaria in pregnancy, and oriented 5,759 health workers on the simplified malaria guidelines. With FY 2013 funding, PMI will fund supportive supervision to ensure that the implementation of the revised IPTp policy among health facility workers is underway. PMI will also strengthen

---

[1] These endemic districts reflect the administrative divisions as of 2009. In 2010, the districts were split into 13 districts. As of 2013, Kenya will be administratively split into 47 counties. The four districts sprayed in 2012 span parts of 3 different counties. This may have some implications on where PMI may spray in 2013 as county governments may be reluctant to spray only part of a county.

community-based behavior change and social mobilization activities that are designed to increase client demand for ANC and IPTp services.

Case management: The third, and most recent, edition of Kenya's national guidelines for diagnosis, treatment and prevention of malaria was issued in 2010, and recommends diagnosis-based treatment as part of effective case management. By the end of 2012, PMI will have procured over two million rapid diagnostic tests (RDTs) as part of its support in rolling out the DOMC's new diagnosis policy of RDT use in all dispensaries and health centers. During the past year, PMI will have also procured an estimated five million treatments of artemether-lumefantrine (AL), cumulating in a total procurement of over 25 million treatments since 2008. With FY 2013 funding, PMI will procure an estimated two million RDTs and support their continued roll-out in malaria endemic areas, as needed, and will support training to strengthen the national reference laboratory. Additionally, PMI will procure over five million treatments of AL to help ensure adequate supply of ACTs in Kenya throughout the year. PMI will also continue to strengthen the supply chain and logistics systems to ensure reliable access and a steady supply of these essential medications. To ensure that AL is properly used and to improve the quality of malaria case management, PMI will help strengthen the DOMC's direct supervision system.

Behavior change communication (BCC): Through community mobilization, interpersonal communication and use of mass media and/or local radio stations to disseminate key messages and encourage correct health seeking behavior, PMI is promoting increased ITN use, prompt diagnosis and treatment for fever, and demand for IPTp in targeted prioritized communities. With FY 2013 funding, PMI will continue to support this cross-cutting BCC investment at community and national levels.

Monitoring and evaluation (M&E): The PMI/Kenya program works to ensure that critical gaps in the DOMC M&E strategy and plan are filled and helps to standardize data collection and reporting. Over the past five years, PMI has supported epidemiology training, *in vivo* antimalarial drug efficacy monitoring, the 2008-09 Demographic and Health Survey, and the 2010 Malaria Indicator Survey. With FY 2013 funds, PMI will support the 2014 MIS survey and continue support to increase the DOMC's M&E capacity to analyze routine data and conduct ongoing program monitoring for specific interventions. These areas of support include: epidemiologic surveillance in IRS districts to inform scale-back timelines and to track epidemics; malaria surveillance in all epidemiological zones; continuous monitoring of malaria in pregnancy activities; monitoring quality of care for malaria case management; and the logistics management information system to monitor commodity stockouts. With FY 2013 funds, PMI will also support collection of malaria information at the district health facility level through the District Health Information System.

Health Systems Strengthening and Integration: In line with GHI principles, PMI has reinforced its efforts to build capacity and integrate across programs. PMI/Kenya strengthens the overall health system by improving governance in the pharmaceutical sector, strengthening pharmaceutical management systems, expanding access to essential medicines, and improving service delivery in the different intervention areas. In 2012, PMI supported the implementation of the malaria commodity logistics management information system, emergency AL distribution to avoid stockouts, and drug quality monitoring. PMI also trained community health workers in focused antenatal care and malaria in pregnancy, supported training and supervision of health workers in IPTp, and trained laboratory technicians in malaria diagnosis. With FY 2013 funds, PMI will continue to work to implement quality assurance and quality control systems for malaria diagnostics. To build human resource capacity and improve service delivery, PMI continues to train health workers at the facility and community levels.

GLOBAL HEALTH INITIATIVE

Malaria prevention and control is a major foreign assistance objective of the U.S. Government (USG). In May 2009, President Barack Obama announced the Global Health Initiative (GHI), a comprehensive effort to reduce the burden of disease and promote healthy communities and families around the world. Through the GHI, the United States will help partner countries improve health outcomes, with a particular focus on improving the health of women, newborns and children. The GHI is a global commitment to invest in healthy and productive lives, building upon and expanding the USG's successes in addressing specific diseases and issues.

The GHI aims to maximize the impact the United States achieves for every health dollar it invests, in a sustainable way. The GHI's business model is based on these key concepts: implementing a woman- and girl-centered approach; increasing impact and efficiency through strategic coordination and programmatic integration; strengthening and leveraging key partnerships, multilateral organizations, and private contributions; encouraging country ownership and investing in country-led plans and health systems; improving metrics, monitoring and evaluation; and promoting research and innovation. The GHI will build on the USG's accomplishments in global health, accelerating progress in health delivery and investing in a more lasting and shared approach through the strengthening of health systems. Framed within the larger context of the GHI and consistent with the GHI's overall principles and planning processes, BEST (Best practices at scale in the home, community and facilities) is a United States Agency for International Development (USAID) planning and review process that draws on our best experience in Family Planning, Mother and Child Health, and Nutrition to base our programs on the best practices to achieve the best impact.

PRESIDENT'S MALARIA INITIATIVE

The President's Malaria Initiative (PMI) is a core component of the GHI, along with HIV/AIDS, maternal and child health, and tuberculosis. PMI was launched in June 2005 as a five-year, $1.2 billion initiative to rapidly scale up malaria prevention and treatment interventions and reduce malaria-related mortality by 50% in 15 high-burden countries in sub-Saharan Africa. With passage of the 2008 Lantos-Hyde Act, funding for PMI has now been extended through FY 2014, and as part of the GHI, the goal of PMI is to achieve a 70% reduction in the burden of malaria in the original 15 countries by 2015. This will be achieved by reaching 85% coverage of the most vulnerable groups — children under five years of age and pregnant women — with proven preventive and therapeutic interventions, including artemisinin-based combination therapies (ACTs), insecticide-treated nets (ITNs), intermittent preventive treatment for pregnant women (IPTp), and indoor residual spraying (IRS).

Kenya was selected as a PMI country in FY 2007. Large-scale implementation of ITNs, ACTs and IPTp began in FY 2008 and has progressed rapidly with support from PMI and other partners. This FY 2013 Malaria Operational Plan (MOP) presents a detailed implementation plan for Kenya, based on the PMI Multi-Year Strategy and Plan, and the Division of Malaria Control's (DOMC) national malaria strategy. It was developed in consultation with the DOMC and with participation of national and international partners involved with malaria prevention and control in the country. The activities that PMI is proposing to support fit in well with the

DOMC's strategic plan and build on investments made by PMI and other partners to improve and expand malaria-related services. This document briefly reviews the current status of malaria control policies and interventions in Kenya, describes progress to date, identifies challenges and unmet needs that must be addressed if the targets of the DOMC and PMI are to be achieved, and provides a description of planned FY 2013 activities.

BACKGROUND

Kenya's 2010 population is approximately 40.5 million people, with an estimated population growth of 2.8% per year.[2] Children under five years of age account for about 16% of the total population.[3] Geographically, the country falls into two main regions: lowland areas, both coastal and around lake basins, and highland areas on both sides of the Great Rift Valley. Kenya has approximately 42 ethnic groups, and is a predominantly agricultural economy with a strong industrial base. Kenya is ranked 143 out of 187 countries on the 2011 United Nation's Human Development Index, which measures life expectancy, adult literacy and per capita income. Life expectancy in Kenya has seen an overall downward trend since the late 1980s, but has recently increased to 56.5 years.[4] The HIV/AIDS estimated adult prevalence is 6%.[5] The total expenditure on health increased from 4.1% of the gross domestic product in 2004 to 7.9% in 2007. The per capita health expenditures in Kenya have also risen from $9 in 2000 to $33 in 2009.[6] There has been a remarkable decline of 36% in under-five child mortality from 115 deaths per 1,000 live births recorded in the 2003 Kenyan demographic and health survey (DHS) to 74 deaths per 1,000 observed in the 2008-09 DHS.[7]

Following the 2010 Constitutional Referendum, Kenya will institute a devolved government, with provinces giving way to 47 counties as the unit of administration in 2013. This change will necessitate the alignment of the implementation of PMI interventions to the new administrative units in 2013. This organizational change may impact operational costs, due to new county-level malaria focal points to equip, train and support the GOK including addressing all other logistical and political pressures.

Ministry of Health
Following the signing of the National Accord and Reconciliation Act of 2008, and as part of the Government's reorganization process, the Ministry of Health was split into the Ministry of Public Health and Sanitation (MOPHS) and the Ministry of Medical Services. The role of MOPHS is to provide focus on public health and preventive measures and leadership in ensuring that public health policy objectives are implemented. The strategic goals and priority investments of each Ministry are designed to ensure that adequate human, infrastructure, and financial resources are available to support program implementation. In addition, within its 2008-2012 Strategic Plan, the MOPHS has a stated goal of "*reducing malaria incidence to 15% through utilization of cost-effective control measures*". Although each of the Ministries has different

---

[2] World Bank, http://data.worldbank.org/country/kenya
[3] 2009 Kenya Population and Housing Census Ibid, page 38
[4] World Bank, http://data.worldbank.org/country/kenya
[5] 2009 Kenya Population and Housing Census Ibid, page 239
[6] WHO Global Health Observatory—Kenya Profile. www.apps.who.int/ghodata last accessed on May 24, 2011
[7] KNBS and IFC Macro, page 129

functions, they work closely together to avoid duplication of efforts. At the central level, both Ministries oversee, govern and facilitate health activities, while passing on more responsibility for service provision and supervision to the province, district, and soon to be county levels. As the new constitution is implemented, it is expected that the two ministries of health will be merged in the near future.

The DOMC is part of the MOPHS, and is staffed by technical professionals who are seconded from other departments and divisions in the ministry. The division has six technical units: vector control, diagnosis and case management, malaria in pregnancy, epidemic preparedness and response, advocacy communication and social mobilization, and surveillance, monitoring and evaluation, and operational research. Each unit has a focal point and one or more technical officers. In 2009, the MOPHS supported a Malaria Program Performance Review, which found that the DOMC was strong in its structure and functioning at the central level, but had a weak coordinating capacity at provincial and district levels. This resulted in a lack of support for the delivery of malaria control interventions as well as for monitoring and evaluation. In late 2012 or early 2013 Kenya is expected to devolve from a national system of governance to a county system of governance. This devolution will likely pose continued challenges to the DOMC in overseeing the country's malaria control program, as the role of the Ministry of Health and the DOMC has yet to be defined.

Figure 1: Map of Kenya

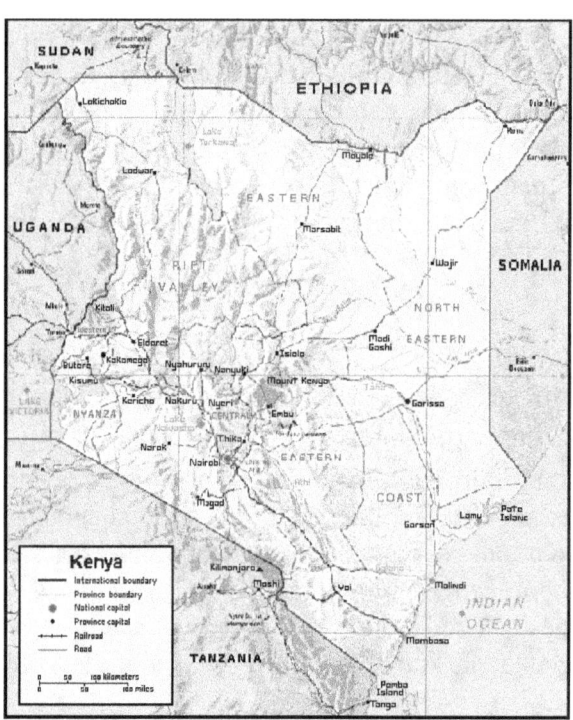

MALARIA SITUATION IN KENYA

Malaria transmission and infection risk in Kenya is determined largely by altitude, rainfall patterns and temperature, and therefore varies considerably across the country and by season. The variations in altitude and terrain create contrasts in the country's climate, which ranges from hot and humid tropical along the coast to temperate in the interior and very dry in the north and northeast. There are two rainy seasons—the long rains occur from April to June and the short rains from October to December. The temperature remains high throughout these months. The hottest period is from February to March and the coldest from July to August. All four species of human *Plasmodium* occur with *Plasmodium falciparum* causing the most severe form of disease and accounting for 98% of all malaria infections. The major malaria vectors are members of the *Anopheles gambiae* complex and *Anopheles funestus.*

About 70% of the population of Kenya is at risk for malaria. The majority of this at-risk population (28 million) lives in areas of low or unstable transmission where *P. falciparum* parasite prevalence is less than 5%. However, an estimated 3.9 million people live in areas of Kenya where parasite prevalence is estimated to be $\geq 40\%$ and malaria remains a serious risk.

For the purposes of malaria control, the country has been stratified into four epidemiological zones:

- **Endemic areas:** These areas of stable malaria have altitudes ranging from 0 to 1,300 meters around Lake Victoria in western Kenya and in the coastal regions[8] of the country. Transmission is intense throughout the year with a *P. falciparum* prevalence between 20%-40% and high annual entomological inoculation rates. Of the total Kenyan population, 29% lives in a malaria endemic zone.

- **Highland epidemic-prone areas:** Malaria transmission in the western highlands is seasonal with considerable year-to-year variation. The entire population is vulnerable and case fatality rates during an epidemic can be up to ten times greater than in endemic regions. Approximately 20% of Kenyans live in these areas; their malaria prevalence ranges from 1% to 5% but with some areas experiencing prevalence between 10% and 20%.

- **Seasonal malaria transmission areas:** This epidemiological zone comprises arid and semi-arid areas of northern and southeastern parts of the country which experience short periods of intense malaria transmission during the rainy seasons. Approximately 21% of the Kenyan population lives within these arid/semi-arid areas of the country; the malaria prevalence is less than 5%.

---

[8] The DOMC is maintaining Coast Province in this zone even though the area has seen a recent decrease in malaria (currently carrying an estimated malaria risk classification of less than 5%). This is because this reduction is not yet stable and the risk for a resurgence of malaria burden in the area remains.

- **Low malaria risk areas:** This zone covers the central highlands of Kenya including Nairobi. Approximately 30% of Kenyans live in these areas where there is little to no disease transmission.

The country's endemicity map (Figure 2 below) was updated in 2009, and depicts the current malaria transmission intensity for the entire country, with high transmission intensity in endemic zones highlighted by the dark shaded areas.

Figure 2: 2009 Kenya Malaria Endemicity Map

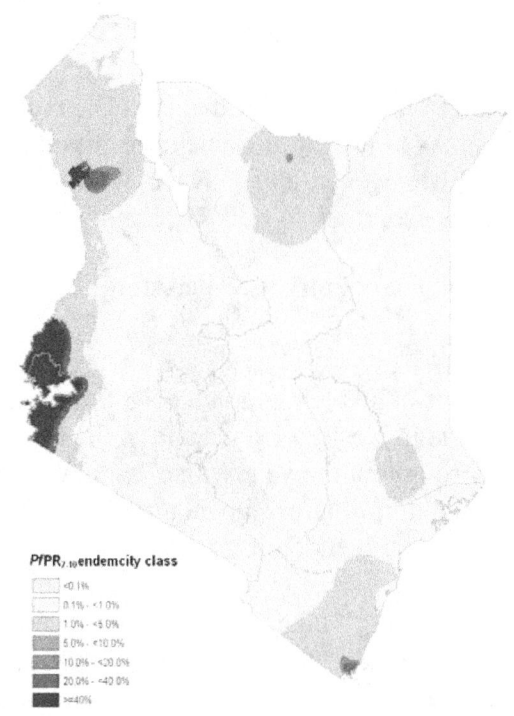

The assembly of limited outpatient and more comprehensive hospital inpatient data[9] provides additional strong evidence that many previous malaria at-risk areas are transitioning towards low, stable transmission conditions.

National Malaria Control Plan and Strategy

The Government of Kenya (GOK) remains committed to improving health service delivery and places a high priority on malaria control. In order to address malaria morbidity and mortality burden in Kenya, the Government has prioritized malaria prevention and treatment interventions and outlined them in the 2009-2017 National Malaria Strategy (NMS), which has six strategic objectives:

---

[9] Snow RW, Okiro EA, Noor AM, Munguti K, Tetteh G, Juma E. *The coverage and impact of malaria intervention in Kenya 2007-2009*. Division of Malaria Control, Ministry of Public Health and Sanitation, December 2009

1) **Objective 1:** By 2013, to have at least 80% of people living in malaria risk areas using appropriate malaria preventive interventions

2) **Objective 2:** To have 100% of fever cases which present to a health worker receive prompt and effective diagnosis and treatment by 2013

3) **Objective 3:** To ensure that all malaria epidemic-prone districts have the capacity to detect and the ability to respond to malaria epidemics annually

4) **Objective 4:** To strengthen surveillance, monitoring and evaluation systems so that key malaria indicators are routinely monitored and evaluated in all at–risk malaria districts by 2011

5) **Objective 5:** To strengthen advocacy, communication and social mobilization capacities for malaria control to ensure that at least 80% of people in areas at risk of malaria have knowledge on prevention and treatment of malaria by 2014

6) **Objective 6:** By 2013, to strengthen capacity in program management in order to achieve malaria programmatic objectives at all levels of the health care system

Strategies to support the achievement of NMS objectives include adopting a multi-sectoral approach to malaria control; decentralizing malaria control operations to the province, district and county (in the near future); tailoring interventions to the prevailing epidemiology; and strengthening the malaria control performance monitoring system. Given the varied and changing malaria epidemiology, Kenya is targeting appropriate intervention measures for specific malaria risk areas. Figure 3, below, compares the changes in Kenya's endemicity map from 2001 to 2009, and notes the shift towards focusing interventions on key geographic areas for the highest impact.

Figure 3: Kenya's Changing Malaria Epidemiology, 2001-2009

Kenya's 2001 Endemicity Map, by key interventions

Kenya's 2009 Endemicity Map, by key interventions

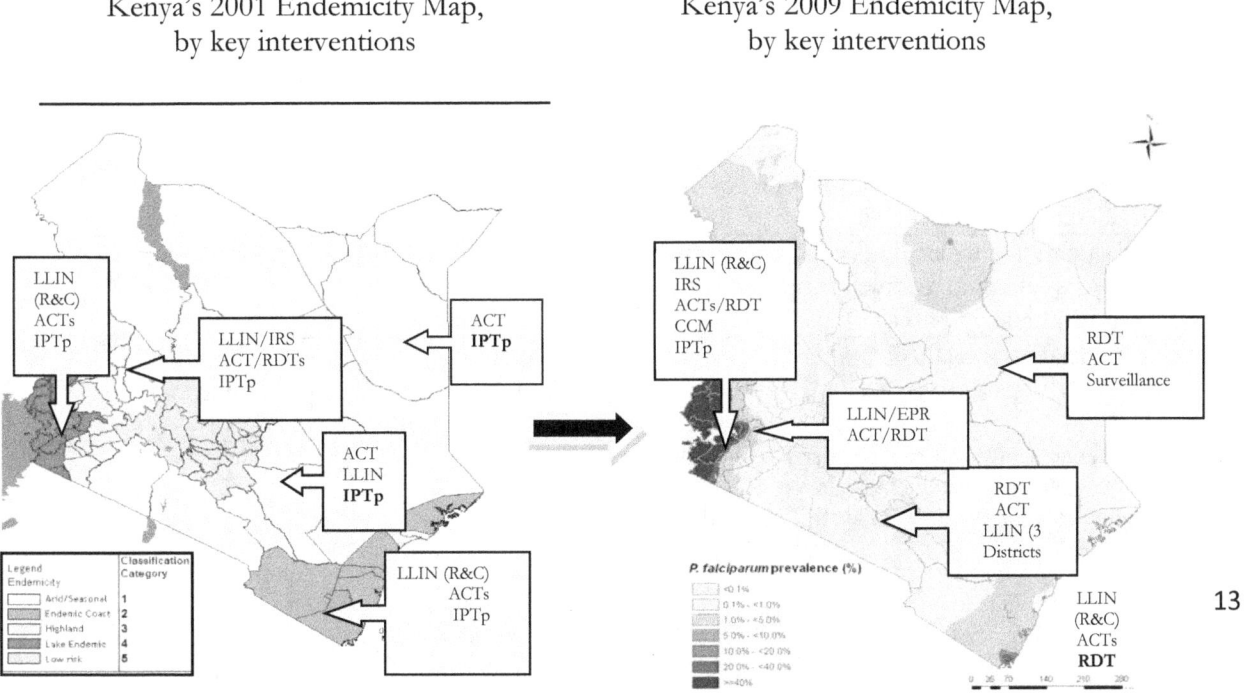

13

The DOMC has strategically reprioritized the approved malaria control interventions according to malaria risk, in order to target resources towards achieving the highest impact possible. Table 1, below, summarizes the interventions targeted by each stratification category.

Table 1: Malaria Interventions, by stratification category

Stratification	CM	ITNs	IRS	IEC/BCC	IPTp	EPR	Surveil-lance
Endemic Areas	X	X	X	X	X		X
Highland Epidemic-Prone Areas	X	X	X	X		X	X
Seasonal Malaria Transmission Areas	X			X		X	X
Low Risk Areas	X			X			X

CURRENT STATUS OF MALARIA INDICATORS

In Kenya, coverage with effective interventions and the ensuing health impact are measured largely through national household surveys. The country proposes to undertake a Malaria Indicator Survey (MIS) once every three years and a DHS once every five years. Routine surveillance through the country's Health Management Information System (HMIS)/District Health Information System (DHIS) and Demographic Surveillance System (DSS) is intended to provide additional data for supplemental analyses. The 2007 MIS and the 2008-09 DHS provided evidence of Kenya's progress in achieving its national targets. Data from the recent 2010 MIS, funded by PMI and the Department for International Development (DfID), has provided updated evidence on the status of key malaria control indicators (Table 2).

Table 2: Summary of Selected Malaria Indicators

	2003 Kenya DHS[i]	2007 Kenya MIS[ii]	2008-09 Kenya DHS[iii]	2010 Kenya MIS
Proportion of households with at least one ITN	6%	48%	56%	48%
Proportion of children under five years old who slept under an ITN the previous night	5%	39%	47%	42%
Proportion of pregnant women who slept under an ITN the previous night	4%	40%	49%	41%
Proportion of women who received two or more doses of sulfadoxine-pyrimethamine (SP) during their last pregnancy in the last two years at least one of which was received during an ANC visit	4%	13%	14%	25%
Proportion of children under five years old with fever in the last two weeks who received treatment with ACTs within 24 hours of onset of fever	N/A	4%	4%	11%
All-cause under-five mortality	115 per 1000 live births	--	74 per 1000 live births	--

[i] Pre-PMI baseline data for all-cause under-five mortality
[ii] PMI baseline data for coverage indicators
[iii] PMI baseline data for all-cause under-five mortality

The 2010 MIS documented minor changes in malaria coverage levels compared to the 2007 baseline.   These indicator changes are described under the various intervention sections below.

MALARIA CONTROL FUNDING SOURCES

Although the DOMC's NMS budget request for the 2013-2014 financial year is approximately $239 million, the available funding to the DOMC, from all sources, for the FY 2013 implementation period (October 2013-September 2014) falls short of the expected need. An analysis of known bilateral and multilateral donors (Table 3) shows that during the period in question (shaded) the confirmed contributors to malaria control will be from Global Fund, DfID and PMI, with the Affordable Medicines Facility-malaria (AMFm) support ending by December 2012 (at the time of writing, the plan for ongoing support for an AMFm subsidy is unknown). Based on this analysis, the PMI Kenya team has concluded that its FY 2013 budget ($32.4 million) will need to fill significant priority gaps, leaving little flexibility to meet less essential yet still important activities. As discussed in the following sections, the FY 2013 budget and activities have been developed in light of available donor funding.

Table 3: Malaria control donor funding & contributions, by calendar year and quarter (shaded quarters indicate when PMI's FY 2013 funding will be available)

Donor Source	2012		2013				2014			
	Q3	Q4	Q1	Q2	Q3	Q4	Q1	Q2	Q3	Q4
Global Fund										
Round 10; Ph1, Yr1	$9.3 million									
Round 10; Ph1, Yr2			$29 million							
Round 10; Ph2, Yr3									TBD	
DfID										
FY 2012	£16.6 million									
FY 2013, (est.)				£15 million						
FY 2014, (est.)									£14.5 million	
PMI										
FY 2011	$36.4 m									
FY 2012		$36.4 million								
FY 2013							$32.4 million			
FY 2014 (est.)										TBD
AMFm *(from GF R 4 funds)*	~32 million ACTs									

Global Fund: The Malaria Round 10 grant covers a five-year period, from October 2011 through September 2016. Phase 1 (ending in December 2013) is valued at $38.4 million for the first two years of implementation. The grant has been scaled back from the initially approved proposal, and it will not fully fund anticipated prevention and treatment needs over the implementation period and additional donor support is needed. While it is intended that the national supply of ACTs will be fully funded by the Global Fund Round 10 grant, the final budget for ACT procurement during Phase 1 (December 2011-December 2013) was negotiated using the current AMFm prices. Since AMFm is scheduled to end in December 2012, and the plans for a continued private sector subsidy have yet to be defined, it is unclear at the time of writing whether or not sufficient funds remain in Phase 1 to fully fund the national ACT needs through the end of 2013 if the subsidy is not continued. Additionally, the planned 2014 ITN mass distribution campaign is not fully funded through the grant and will need to be supported by additional donor funds in order to be fully implemented.

DfID: The UK's Department for International Development (DfID) has renewed its commitment to supporting malaria control in Kenya for another five years (2011-2015). The new strategy allocates £58.4 million for malaria programming and is intended to: continue to support the distribution of free ITNs through antenatal care (ANC) clinics (£32m), strengthen Kenya's vector control efforts as outlined in the DOMC's malaria strategy (£5m), and add support for IRS programs and strengthening of the country's malaria information systems (£21m). This malaria investment is part of a large scale-up of DfID's international public health funding, currently estimated to be up to £510 million over the five-year strategy. This expanded support for the malaria control program and the health sector overall is still being developed, and PMI is working closely with DfID staff to identify how these new investments may complement those of PMI. Of particular interest is DfID's planned expansion into the IRS program, which will be a timely and welcome investment as Kenya is likely to shift its program to a non-pyrethroid insecticide which will greatly increase the operational costs of the program (discussed further in the IRS section, below). As of writing, the DfID budget for the 2013/2014 fiscal year, which overlaps with the PMI fiscal year discussed in this MOP, is estimated to be £15 million, including the procurement of 1.225 million ITNs for distribution through the routine system. DfID is expected to finalize its plans and confirm budget figures in early 2013.

Affordable Medicines Facility—Malaria (AMFm): The funding for the AMFm proposal is from the Global Fund's Round 4 grant, which had a budget of $18,329,872 for ACT procurement. These funds were reprogrammed to support AMFm interventions, with approximately $2 million designated for ACT procurement using the AMFm subsidized price structure. With this level of funding, approximately 12 million ACTs (including 1.1 million ACTs for community-level distribution) were procured in 2011. An additional 11 million ACTs were procured and distributed to public sector facilities in 2012. Implementation of the AMFm was from June 2010-December 2012. As of writing, it is not yet known how the AMFm subsidy program will continue after December 2012. As noted above (and discussed further in the case management section below) this may have significant consequences for the stability of Kenya's public sector supply of ACTs.

World Bank: While no new World Bank funding is available for malaria control support in Kenya, the World Bank did reprogram some of its existing funding to procure 2.3 million ITNs for the 2012 universal coverage campaign for Coast Province.

EXPECTED RESULTS—YEAR SIX (FY 2013)

Prevention:
1. Proportion of pregnant women in targeted areas who receive two or more doses of IPTp during their pregnancy will have increased to 50%
2. Proportion of households with at least one ITN will have increased to 70%
3. Proportion of pregnant women sleeping under an ITN the previous night will have increased to 60%
4. 95% of houses in geographic areas targeted for IRS will have been sprayed.

Treatment:
1. Proportion of government health facilities with ACTs available for treatment of uncomplicated malaria will increase to 100%
2. Proportion of children under five years old with fever in the last two weeks who had a finger or heel stick will have increased from 12% (2010 MIS) to 50%.

PREVENTION ACTIVITIES

Insecticide-Treated Nets

Background

Under the 2009-2017 Kenya NMS, one of the objectives of the DOMC is to attain universal coverage of ITNs, defined as reaching a ratio of one ITN for every two people, in conjunction with increasing use of those nets to 80%, within prioritized regions of the country by 2013. Universal coverage is to be achieved through multiple distribution channels including mass distribution of ITNs to all households in the targeted regions every three years, routine distribution to all pregnant women and children under one year, and social marketing of nets at subsidized prices in targeted markets. The national specifications for ITN products are currently being revised, and should be finalized by December 2012. Funding from the Global Fund Round 10 malaria grant, in combination with significant contributions from other donors, will enable Kenya to maintain national coverage targets through the following distribution strategies (summarized in Table 4, below):

Mass Distribution: The 2011-2012 mass ITN distribution campaign, which will provide over 20 million people with access to free ITNs, should reach the country's universal coverage targets by December 2012. The DOMC quantifies the LLIN needs for a mass distribution campaign by dividing the targeted population by 1.8, as recommended by the WHO. In 2011, this rolling campaign distributed over 7.6 million ITNs to Western, Nyanza and targeted parts of Rift Valley Provinces. In 2012, the national campaign will be completed with a distribution of an estimated three million ITNs in Coast Province. The DOMC plans to conduct mass distribution campaigns in targeted endemic and epidemic-prone districts every three years, and estimates that for the next campaign, planned for 2014, about 12 million nets will be needed to maintain universal coverage in endemic and epidemic-prone districts in Nyanza, Western, Rift Valley and Coast Provinces. There are enough funds in the Global Fund Round 10 grant to cover approximately

60% of the 2014 mass distribution replacement campaign, while the balance of support will need to come from partners (such as PMI).

Continuous Distribution with Public Sector ITNs: Currently, the DOMC continues to support routine distribution of free ITNs to pregnant women and children through ANC and child welfare clinics. Routine distribution is targeted for all vulnerable populations living in all malaria endemic and epidemic-prone areas in Kenya, and exceeds the geographic areas targeted in the mass distribution campaign. It remains the primary channel for access to ITNs between mass distribution campaigns. In anticipation of reaching universal ITN coverage by the end of 2012 and striving to maintain it after the 2014 replacement campaign, a key challenge for Kenya will be developing a systematic way of replacing worn-out nets among targeted households. Developing a comprehensive continuous distribution system to replace nets in targeted households in a cost effective manner is a critical step in maintaining high coverage levels and removing the need for mass distribution campaigns over the long run.

Social Marketing in the Private Sector: Through its support to a private sector partner, Population Services International, DfID has supported a small social marketing program, which sells about 500,000 ITNs per year on the open market. These ITNs sell for KSH 50 (~USD $0.60) each and are primarily sold in rural areas in endemic and epidemic-prone districts. The DOMC estimates that demand for socially marketed nets exceeds current supply levels, and is a program that could be expanded.

Private Sector Commercial Sales: While the national policy supports only the distribution and sale of ITNs, local manufacturers are still producing untreated nets. Previously, Population Services International, with DfID support, has bundled some of these locally manufactured nets with a long-lasting retreatment kit and is selling them at a subsidized price through its retail outlets. However, Population Services International does not have funding to continue this activity and is in discussions with the DOMC and local manufacturers to try to ensure that locally-produced nets continue to be bundled with insecticide, to ensure that these conventional nets are in accordance with national policy. The DOMC supports strategies to promote a sustainable ITN market, including decreased taxes and tariffs on netting material and development and airing of generic demand-creation messages from which manufacturers can promote their individual brands.

Table 4: National ITN Distribution Strategies, by approach

	Target Population	Target Areas	Method	Current Donors
Universal coverage via mass distribution	One ITN for every two people	Priority malaria endemic and epidemic-prone provinces (Western, Nyanza, Rift Valley and Coast)	Free of charge	Global Fund, World Bank, World Vision, PMI
Routine distribution to ANC and child welfare clinics	Pregnant women and children under one	Endemic, epidemic and seasonal transmission districts	Free of charge	DfID, PMI
Routine distribution to comprehensive care clinics	HIV/AIDS infected persons	Nationwide, but prioritized by HIV/AIDS endemic provinces	Free of charge	PEPFAR and Global Fund
Commercial sector sales	Those who can afford commercially priced nets	Urban/rural centers	Imported ITNs sold at full cost (USD$7-10) in urban shops.	Financed by private sector
Social marketing to communities	Households in targeted areas	Rural areas in priority malaria endemic and epidemic-prone provinces	ITNs sold for KSH 50 ($0.60) at health clinics	DfID

ITN Coverage and Use: Data from MIS and DHS surveys over the past decade have shown considerable progress in access to ITNs. ITN ownership increased from 6% in 2003 to 48% in 2007 following a targeted mass distribution campaign. With consistent support for routine distribution through ANCs, the 2010 MIS results document that household ownership of at least one ITN remained at 48%. Likewise, the ITN use among pregnant women (41%) and children under five (42%) has also remained stable from the 2007 MIS baseline (where use was ~40% for both target groups). The MIS found that in 2010, the ITN ownership ratio was one ITN for every five people at risk in Kenya. While the ITN coverage levels have not increased since 2007, given that over 10 million nets were distributed in 2011 and 2012 (after the data for the MIS was collected), the DOMC expects that ITN ownership has increased dramatically since the 2010 MIS, which will be reflected during the next national household survey. PMI supported a post-campaign survey to understand the effectiveness of the campaign on ITN ownership and use. Preliminary analysis suggests that low levels of ITN use are a major barrier to maximizing the public health benefits from universal coverage, and may necessitate a more intensive effort to promote the correct and consistent use of ITNs. The data continue to be analyzed, and final results are expected to be released by October 2012.

ITN Gap Analysis: As detailed below, the ITN gap analysis for FY 2013 highlights the risk associated with anticipated net loss following mass distribution. By 2014, PMI estimates that among the at-risk population living in malaria endemic provinces who qualify for universal ITN coverage, there will be a 2.7 million ITN gap, based on the estimated population growth and the national policy to fully replace nets 36 months after distribution. For the routine distribution system, based on pledged ITNs from PMI and DfID, PMI anticipates that the routine system needs will be met.

Table 5: FY 2013 ITN Gap Analysis Table

A. Targeted Campaign Districts (endemic districts in Western, Nyanza and Coast)

Data Inputs	Country data
At-Risk Population (2010 Estimates)	20,250,000
Expected annual population growth	2.80%
Average number of persons per net	1.8
Distributed ITNs	
Distributed ITNs in 2011 (UC Campaign only)	7,600,000
Distributed ITNs in 2012 to date (UC Campaign only)	0
ITNs pledged to be distributed in 2012 (UC Campaign only)	3,000,000
Pledged ITNs	
ITNs pledged to be distributed in 2013 (UC Campaign only)	0
ITNs pledged to be distributed in 2014 (UC Campaign only, includes)	~7,200,000

2014 Campaign ITNs Need Calculation

Population at risk in 2014 (UC Campaign Districts)	21,399,876
Total number of ITNs needed (UC Campaign Districts only)	12,221,707
Viable Nets from Previous years (3 year durability, UC Campaign Districts). *(Assumes 20% ITN loss at 24 months post distribution and that all nets older than 36 months should be replaced))*	2,400,000
Total Estimated Available Nets in-country	7,200,000
ITN gap	**2,621,707**

B. ANC/EPI Routine Distribution (for pregnant women and children under one)

Population at risk in 2014 (Routine System)	2,901,581
Total number of ITNs needed (Routine System)	2,901,581
Viable Nets from Previous years	0
Pledged ITNs	
Pledged ITNs in 2014 (via routine distribution) (includes pledged ITNs from: PMI: 1,300,000; and DfID: 1,500,000)	2,800,000
ITN gap	**101,581**
Data Source: 2010 Global Fund Round 10 Kenya Proposal	

Progress to Date

Routine Distribution: PMI continues to support the DOMC's routine distribution program, to ensure that vulnerable populations (pregnant women and children under one) have consistent access to ITNs. With FY 2011 funding, PMI procured 1.3 million ITNs for distribution through the routine system, building upon previous investments in this channel. An estimated 300,000 ITNs will be distributed by September 2012, and the balance is scheduled to be distributed by early 2013. PMI continues to partner with DfID to ensure that 100% of the ITN needs for distribution through the routine system are fully met.

Universal Coverage Mass Distribution: In support of the 2011 Phase 1 mass campaign, PMI procured and distributed over 2.5 million nets for priority districts in Western, Nyanza and Rift Valley Provinces, representing 33% of the 7.6 million nets distributed during this campaign. PMI also supported the campaign's logistic costs and a post-campaign survey, which informed the revision of the planning and procedures for the mass campaign in Coast Province in 2012. Preliminary results from the post-campaign survey showed that ITN use remained low following the campaign (final results are expected by October 2012). Therefore, PMI continues to promote increased use of ITNs distributed through both the universal coverage campaign as well as through the routine system, (i.e., through national and community-based communication activities as discussed in detail in the BCC section).

In summary, as of the end of FY 2012, after five years of implementation, PMI will have purchased a total of over 5.2 million ITNs and distributed an estimated 3.8 million ITNs in both mass campaigns and routine distribution efforts – making a significant contribution towards the overall ITN coverage rate in the country.

Proposed PMI Activities with FY 2013 Funding: *($10,200,000)*

1. *Procure and distribute ITNs for Routine Distribution and the 2014 Mass Distribution Campaign*:
   - *Routine Distribution:* Fill 50% of the ITN gap for routine distribution by purchasing 1.3 million ITNs to distribute free-of-charge to pregnant women and children under one through the ANC and child welfare clinics. *($5,850,000)*
   - *2014 Mass Distribution:* Support the scheduled 2014 mass distribution campaign to sustain universal coverage in high priority malaria endemic areas by procuring approximately 500,000 ITNs. *($2,250,000)*

2. *Logistics and Program Support for Routine and Mass Campaign Distribution:* Provide logistical support, including transportation and storage of nets, for distribution of the 1.8 million ITNs both within the national routine distribution system and for the 2014 mass campaign. *($1,800,000)*

3. *Strengthen the Continuous Distribution System:* Continue strengthening Kenya's continuous ITN distribution system to maintain the universal coverage levels achieved in 43 priority districts in the aftermath of the mass distribution campaign. This activity will

seek to identify and close distribution gaps and promote cost-effective tracking systems to ensure that populations living in targeted districts will be able to replace ITNs as they wear out, with the ultimate goal of ending the need for mass campaigns to keep ITN coverage at optimal levels. *($300,000)*

4. *Behavior change for correct and consistent use of ITNs:* Support and expand targeted community BCC and social mobilization to increase demand for and uptake of ITNs. Messages and mode of dissemination will be dependent on the venue and target group. Interpersonal communication will be used in health facilities and the ANC clinics for patients, in homes during home visits by community health workers, and at *Barazas* in villages and during public gatherings where messages are delivered through public address systems. *(This activity is budgeted under the BCC section)*

5. *Technical assistance:* Support one visit from USAID to provide technical assistance for the implementation of the ITN program. *(Core funded)*

Indoor Residual Spraying

Background

Through 2010, the DOMC's IRS program targeted sixteen highland, epidemic-prone districts in Western Kenya. As ITN coverage has expanded throughout Kenya, malaria prevalence has fallen sharply, particularly in those highland districts that had been targeted for IRS activities. Both the Global Fund Round 4 malaria grant and PMI funded IRS campaigns in the highland districts, with PMI providing concentrated technical assistance and capacity building.

With the 2009-2017 Kenya NMS, the DOMC has phased out IRS in the highland, epidemic-prone districts and begun to focus on endemic districts, particularly those bordering the highlands. According to the national strategy, IRS should be implemented for at least three years while ITNs are scaled up to achieve universal coverage, after which IRS may be phased out. Beginning in May of 2010, the PMI-supported IRS program expanded to cover three lowland districts[10] along Lake Victoria which border highland, epidemic-prone districts. In 2012, PMI-supported IRS operations were expanded to a total of four lowland districts. These districts are located in areas with some of the highest *P. falciparum* prevalence rates in the country. While PMI is currently the only partner supporting IRS campaigns in these important lowland districts, DfID is developing plans to support further expansion of IRS campaigns to other areas around the lake. The DfID program is expected to begin in late 2013.

Through 2012, IRS was conducted using pyrethroid insecticides. Pyrethroid resistance had been detected in *An. gambiae* s.s. in western Kenya but this species was significantly reduced by ITNs and was largely absent in the districts targeted for IRS. This species was most common in areas

---

[10] These endemic districts reflect the administrative divisions as of 2009. In 2010, the original three districts were split into 10 districts while the fourth district sprayed in 2012 was split into three districts. As of 2013, Kenya will be administratively split into 47 counties. The four districts sprayed in 2012 span parts of three different counties. This may have some implications on where PMI may spray in 2013 as county governments may be reluctant to spray only part of a county.

near the Ugandan border. As of late 2012, however, the range of *An. gambiae* s.s. was expanding eastward. Furthermore, pyrethroid resistance was observed in *An. arabiensis* in the district that had been sprayed for four consecutive years. Given the increasing pyrethroid resistance in western Kenya, the DOMC has advocated a shift from one annual round of IRS with pyrethroids to two annual rounds with carbamates. This change in policy will have important implications for the size of the target population that can be covered and it is likely that IRS will need to cease in some areas that have been receiving it.

With IRS efforts shifting away from the highlands, the DOMC has moved to an epidemic surveillance and response system to detect rising cases of malaria and respond using a combination of targeted IRS and improved case management. The details of this are described in the section on Epidemic Surveillance and Response.

Progress to Date

The PMI IRS program in Kenya began in 2008. PMI spraying was done in conjunction with the Kenya DOMC which conducted IRS in focal areas in sixteen highland districts. PMI assumed responsibility for spraying two highland districts aiming for complete coverage. In addition, PMI sprayed one lowland endemic district that bordered the highlands as an initial phase of plans to create a buffer between the lowland endemic districts and the highland epidemic districts where IRS was slated to be phased out. PMI sprayed the same three districts in 2009.

In the 2010 spray round, the DOMC assumed responsibility for IRS in the highlands while PMI supported IRS in three lowland districts including the lowland district that had been previously sprayed by PMI in 2008 and 2009. The same three lowland districts were sprayed in 2011 and 2012. A fourth lowland district was sprayed for the first time in 2012. To date, all IRS in Kenya has been conducted using pyrethroid insecticides. The target populations and annual spray coverages are provided in the table below:

Table 6: PMI IRS Program Coverage, 2008-2012

Year	Districts	Targeted Households	Targeted Population	Coverage
2008	2 highland, 1 lowland	764,050	3,061,967	96%
2009	2 highland, 1 lowland	517,051	1,435,272	94.6%
2010	3 lowland	503,707	1,892,725	97.1%
2011	3 lowland	485,043	1,832,090	89%
2012*	4 lowland	692,258	2,189,275	98%
*Preliminary estimates				

PMI and other donors provided support for surveillance and monitoring to document the effectiveness of IRS in areas with high ITN coverage after the 2008 and 2009 spray rounds. While these initial surveys indicated a reduction in the incidence of parasitemia and the prevalence of parasitemia and anemia. More recent national data from the 2010 MIS suggest that malaria prevalence in these areas remains high in spite of multiple interventions, including the scale-up of ITNs. While IRS is expected to reduce the malaria prevalence burden in the targeted districts, heightened surveillance is needed to monitor progress. Surveillance will become more important as IRS operations and their geographic coverage are scaled back due to the increased cost associated with switching from one annual spray round with pyrethroids to two annual rounds with a carbamate insecticide.

The switch in insecticides from pyrethroids to carbamates is necessitated by the emergence of insecticide resistance throughout much of western Kenya. Insecticide resistance monitoring has been conducted at eight sites in western Kenya. As of 2010, moderate to high levels of DDT and pyrethroid resistance were initially detected in *An. gambiae* s.s. in sites near the Uganda border. Observed resistance in this species has ranged from 38 to 67% for DDT, 72 to 84% for permethrin and 37 to 58% for deltamethrin. However, *An. gambiae* was rare or even absent in sites along the lake shore, including the districts where PMI has been conducting IRS operations. In late 2011, *An. gambiae* increased in frequency in areas further from the Uganda border. Furthermore, pyrethroid resistance was observed in several districts in western Kenya, including two of the IRS districts where *An. arabiensis* has been the predominant vector. Data from a PMI-supported operational research study showed the best alternative was a bendiocarb (a carbamate) based on acceptability and duration of efficacy. Given the increased operational costs associated with using non-pyrethroid insecticides, this decision is likely to have significant impact on the geographic coverage and the total population protected by future IRS programs. Figure 4, below, shows pyrethroid resistance in *An. gambiae* s.l. in districts in western Kenya, including three districts that were sprayed by PMI (Migori, Nyando & Rachuonyo). Insecticides should be changed if more than 20% of mosquitoes are determined to be resistant in WHO tube bioassays.

Figure 4: Pyrethroid Insecticide Resistance in Kenya (2011), by targeted district

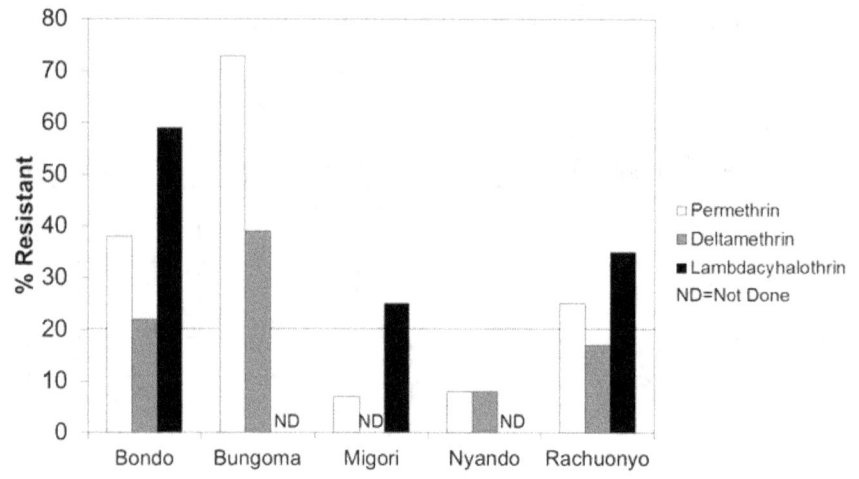

Proposed PMI Activities with FY 2013 Funding: *($7,192,400)*

With FY 2013 funding, PMI will spray up to three endemic districts. PMI will also provide support to the DOMC to monitor disease trends in districts where IRS is phased out. Specific activities include:

1. *IRS implementation:* Support two rounds of IRS with a carbamate in up to three endemic districts with a target of 85% coverage in all districts. The geographic targets will be decided in consultation with the DOMC as well as the county governments that will be formed under the new constitution. The exact target population will depend on the exact cost for spraying with the new insecticide. Based on the cost of the insecticide and the need for two rounds of spraying, we estimate that the population covered will be 346,000 households with a total population of 1.1 million. *($7,000,000)*

2. *Facility-based epidemiological surveillance:* Support facility-based epidemiological surveillance and monitoring in endemic IRS districts to provide information that the DOMC can use to make decisions on the best strategy for IRS. The health facility-based disease burden monitoring is designed to monitor malaria burden over time and to provide the DOMC with data that will guide the scale-down of IRS in the wake of universal ITN coverage. (*This activity is budgeted under the M&E section*)

3. *Entomological monitoring:* Given the expansion of IRS in lowland areas of western Kenya, the detection of low levels of insecticide resistance in border areas near Uganda and the recent expansion eastward, PMI will continue entomologic and insecticide resistance monitoring in eight sites in western Kenya. With additional funding through the DOMC, the number of sites will be expanded to over 40 for 2012 to assist with planning of IRS operations for the future. Monitoring will include determination of species and abundance, insecticide resistance testing and determination of the duration of efficacy of insecticides sprayed on walls. *($180,000)*

4. *Technical assistance:* Support one visit from Centers for Disease Control and Prevention (CDC) to provide technical assistance in the entomological monitoring of IRS activities. *($12,400)*

Malaria in Pregnancy

Background

Kenya's malaria in pregnancy (MIP) program is based on a close working relationship between the Division of Reproductive Health and the DOMC. The Division of Reproductive Health manages program implementation, while the DOMC is responsible for technical oversight. Prevention of MIP is an integral component of the focused antenatal care (FANC) approach in Kenya. The 2008-2009 DHS showed that 92% of women in Kenya receive antenatal care from a medical professional during pregnancy; however, only 15% of women obtain care in the first trimester. Overall, only 47% of pregnant women make four or more antenatal visits during pregnancy, with the median gestational age at first visit being 5.7 months.

The 2009-2017 NMS has a 2013 target of 80% of people living in malaria risk areas using appropriate malaria prevention interventions, however the uptake of IPTp in Kenya has remained low. The results from the most recent 2008-2009 DHS indicate approximately 34% of women who had a live birth in the preceding two years received any sulfadoxine-pyrimethamine (SP) dose during an ANC visit. Whereas the proportion of pregnant women receiving the recommended two or more doses of SP for intermittent preventive treatment of malaria in pregnancy increased from 14% in 2008-9 to 25% in 2010 (KDHS, 2008-2009 and MIS, 2010). While ANC visits provide an opportunity for administration of IPTp doses, additional approaches including a focus on community-based MIP activities began with PMI support in 2011. These activities include MIP messaging, use of community data collection tools to capture IPTp uptake, and referral of pregnant women to health facilities to access IPTp services.

The first-line treatment for malaria in pregnancy is oral quinine in the first trimester of pregnancy and artemether-lumefantrine (AL) or oral quinine in the second and third trimesters. The DOMC recommends diagnosis by blood smear. It also recommends that pregnant women receive ferrous sulfate (200mcg) and folic acid (5mg) at their second and third ANC visits, and that signs and symptoms of anemia are evaluated during their first and fourth ANC visits.

The revised National Guidelines for the Diagnosis, Treatment and Prevention of Malaria in Kenya (May 2010) emphasize the integration of MIP in the overall antenatal care package for maternal health that includes IPTp, LLINs, prompt diagnosis and treatment of fever due to malaria, and health education.

IPTp with SP has been a policy in Kenya since 1998. According to the national guidelines:

- IPTp is recommended in areas of high malaria transmission
- IPTp should be administered with each scheduled visit after quickening to ensure that women receive a minimum of two doses of SP
- IPTp should be given at an interval of at least four weeks
- IPTp should be given under directly observed therapy
- Folic acid tablets should only be administered 14 days following the administration of IPTp

The 2008-09 DHS showed 49% of women and 47% of children under five in Kenya slept under an LLIN the night preceding the interview. While Nyanza and North Eastern Provinces had the highest percentage of children using nets, pregnant women in Coast, Western and North Eastern Provinces showed the highest level of net use. In FY 2013 PMI will support the need for routine distribution of LLINs by purchasing up to 1.8 million LLINs. Mass campaigns and routine distribution will be free of charge to pregnant women and children under one through the ANC and child welfare care clinics to increase the use of LLINs.

In 2008 and 2009, PMI supported the DOMC in a pilot to measure the impact of simplified policy guidelines on MIP to health workers in three malaria endemic districts to improve the uptake of IPTp. The results from the pilot documented the successful nature of the new guidelines that increased the uptake of IPTp among ANC attendees. The process involved orientation of members of the District Health Management Teams (DHMTs) on the IPTp guidelines with an emphasis on administering IPTp during each ANC visit after quickening unless SP had been taken in the prior four weeks. Building on the distribution of the new MIP guidelines, new MIP basic and technical modules were developed to be incorporated into community health workers (CHW) curriculum. The dissemination of simplified messaging and guidelines focuses on service providers in MCH clinics and the training of CHWs. In addition to the continued support to service providers there is a new focus to strengthen activities that support community-based MIP activities through the use of CHWs to create awareness to drive IPTp uptake in 12 select districts. The CHWs will have the capacity to promote the uptake of IPTp at the community level with the capability to trace and refer women who default on treatment.

In addition to ongoing distribution, MIP guidelines are currently being translated into several local languages including Swahili, Luhya, and Luo. There will be a continued focus to expand community-based IEC and BCC efforts by increasing outreach to women and young children via appropriate strategies and channels of communication. Messages and modes of dissemination will be dependent on the venue and target group. Interpersonal communication will be used in hospitals and at ANC clinics, as well as in homes during home visits by CHWs, while *Barazas* will be held in villages and during public gatherings where messages are delivered through public address systems. Finally, there has been an accelerated implementation strategy of the MIP intervention in Bondo District via mentorship on MIP in 17 high-volume health facilities.

In areas with moderate to high malaria transmission, the progress made in the last decade is now under threat from increasing resistance of the parasite to SP, the only antimalarial currently recommended for IPTp. Western Kenya has moderate to high levels of SP resistance, experiencing a dramatic increase in dihydrofolate reductase (*dhfr*) and dihydropteroate synthase (*dhps*) quintuple mutations that confer clinically relevant levels of parasite resistance among pregnant women, from 7% in 1997 to 89% in 2009 (Ya Ping Shi, unpublished data). This has implications for the current policy of using SP for IPTp in endemic areas including Western Province.

The ongoing roll-out of approximately 500,000 RDTs, starting in 2011, is an effective strategy to establish diagnosis of malaria. With the increased availability of malaria RDTs, and the observed reductions in malaria transmission in many parts of Kenya, screening for infection is a key feature of malaria control in pregnancy. In the context of increased SP resistance and decreasing transmission, intermittent screening and treatment in pregnancy (ISTp) provides an alternative strategy for women protected by ITNs. ISTp consists of scheduled screening using a malaria RDT three or four times during pregnancy as part of FANC, and treating RDT-positive women with a long-acting ACT for symptomatic malaria in the second and third trimesters. The previous evidence from a single trial in Ghana, conducted in an area that had low levels of SP resistance, supports ISTp as an effective strategy for areas with low or markedly reduced levels of transmission. PMI will be supporting this activity with FY 2012 funding. The results from this activity are expected to inform national policy on MIP.

Progress to Date

The Kenya Government has been procuring SP for IPTp. In 2011 an estimated 2,000 CHWs were trained on FANC/MIP in Nyanza and Western Provinces. In 2010/2011 there were 39,498 women in 12 districts in Nyanza and Western Provinces who were reached with information on the prevention and treatment of malaria through community BCC activities. PMI continues to support IEC and BCC at the community level for prevention of malaria in pregnancy. PMI support also ensures strengthened monitoring of MIP, including ensuring improved reporting.

PMI continues to support strengthening MIP efforts throughout priority districts. In 2011, PMI supported the production and dissemination of 3,000 guidelines with simplified messages on FANC/MIP to health providers in 64 malaria endemic districts reaching an estimated 5,795 health workers of a targeted 4,940 of whom 3,303 were male and 2,456 were female. A total of 1,165 health facilities were reached as health workers in each were oriented on the simplified guidelines. The simplified messages and guidelines continue to be rolled out in all districts in Western, Nyanza and Coast Provinces in line with the national strategy of targeting IPTp in endemic areas with a focus on supportive supervision.The guidelines will also be used as part of the supportive supervision to reinforce the messaging on IPTp. Health worker skills are being strengthened through the use of the Standards-Based Management and Recognition (SBM-R) approach which seeks to improve standards in quality health care. Plans are underway to review and programmatically evaluate the outcomes of the orientations with the simplified guidelines.

Proposed PMI activities with FY 2013 Funding: *($450,000)*

With FY 2013 funding, PMI will continue to support improving MIP activities. Specific activities include:

1. *IPTp supportive supervision in target endemic districts:* Building on PMI's efforts to roll out the simplified IPTp guidelines, PMI will continue to fund supportive supervision for the trained MCH service providers and CHWs who will have been sensitized on the simplified messaging on IPTp. An estimated 5,759 MCH service providers will be supervised to consolidate gains that will have been achieved through the more intensive FY 2012 investments. The supervision will focus on reinforcing provider skills to improve IPTp2 uptake. In addition, PMI support will continue scale-up of MIP community interventions in 12 districts in Nyanza and Western Provinces. This will include development of the community MIP roll-out plan to be shared with District Health Management Teams (DHMTs) and partners in these provinces. The roll-out of the community component of MIP will include training community MIP trainers of trainers and facilitation of the community MIP TOTs to train 200 Community Health Extension Workers (CHEWs) on community MIP messaging and use of the community data collection tools. The CHEWs will hold monthly consultative meetings to receive data from CHWs. The CHEWs will be facilitated to identify and register pregnant women at the community, trace and refer pregnant women who have not completed IPTp to facilities, attend dialogue days to disseminate MIP messages and attend monthly consultative meetings to review data with CHEWs. CHWs will offer support and work closely with the health facilities to provide SP and other MIP services. It is expected that these community-based activities will ensure increased use of IPTp among pregnant women in the target areas. *($450,000)*

2. *Procure LLIN for routine distribution:* Support the distribution of LLINs free of charge for pregnant women through ANC visits. *(This activity is budgeted under the LLIN section)*

3. *Malaria in pregnancy monitoring and evaluation:* Support monitoring and evaluating the IPTp2 uptake in targeted endemic districts by the DHMTs and DOMC. This will include specific monitoring of the supportive supervision activity such as the quality of supervision provided and health provider perceptions and practice. At the end of the intervention, an evaluation will be undertaken to determine the uptake of IPTp2 among pregnant women. This will provide programmatic information to the DOMC to guide continued implementation of IPTp. The evaluation of the impact of this rolled-out MIP activity funded with the FY 2013 MOP funds will be the last evaluation planned for this activity, as after this point it will be standard GoK policy and fully implemented. The information generated from this activity will be used to inform the program and improve IPTp2 uptake to the target 80% in all target malaria endemic areas. (*This activity is budgeted under the M&E section*)

4. *Behavior change for malaria in pregnancy:* Support and expand targeted community BCC and social mobilization to increase demand for and uptake of IPTp. Messages and mode of dissemination will be dependent on the venue and target group. In health facilities (at the ANC clinics) interpersonal communication will be used as well as in homes during home visits by community health workers, while *Barazas* will be held in villages and during public gatherings where messages are delivered through public address systems. *(This activity is budgeted under the BCC section)*

CASE MANAGEMENT

As part of the overall effort to achieve malaria elimination in Kenya, a key objective of the 2009-2017 NMS is to have at least 80% of self-managed fever cases receive prompt and effective treatment by 2013. Furthermore, the DOMC's target and strategy for case management is to ensure by 2013 that 100% of all fever cases receive a parasitological diagnosis (through microscopy or RDT) and effective treatment. In support of this objective, there is a national commitment to ensure that ACTs are accessible at all public health care levels, including through community health workers, and in the private sector through subsidy schemes. The scaling up of programs, beginning with mass roll-outs of RDTs that started in 2011, have resulted in an increased need for and emphasis on laboratory diagnosis for all age groups presenting with clinical symptoms of malaria at all levels of the health system and in all epidemiological zones.

Malaria Diagnosis

Background

Following adoption of a laboratory diagnosis-based malaria treatment policy, the DOMC produced a third revision of the National Guidelines for Diagnosis, Treatment, and Prevention of Malaria in Kenya. Although the most up-to-date guidelines recommend that the diagnosis of malaria in public health facilities should be based on the detection of parasites in the blood, it stresses that under no circumstances should a patient with suspected malaria be denied treatment, nor should treatment be delayed for lack of a parasitological diagnosis. It also encourages clinicians to confirm malaria even after presumptive treatment has been administered.

In order to achieve the goal of 100% testing of fever cases, in 2011 the DOMC began a nationwide RDT roll-out strategy, beginning with distribution of RDTs to low-risk, epidemic-prone areas and continuing with endemic areas. Because the DOMC's treatment guidelines call for RDTs to be used as the primary method of malaria diagnosis at dispensaries and health centres, the initial distributions have and will continue to be to these facilities. While microscopy remains the gold standard for diagnosis at sub-district, district, provincial and national referral hospitals, the DOMC has begun to procure and distribute RDTs for use in these same facilities, when microscopy is not feasible. RDTs will not be provided to CHWs at the community level until 2013, by which time the DOMC anticipates that dispensaries and health centres will be stocking and properly using RDTs and will function not only as referral centers for CHWs at community level but also be able to properly supervise malaria diagnosis by CHWs.

To facilitate the introduction of RDTs in Kenya, an RDT implementation pilot was conducted in 2012 to measure the impact of RDT use on malaria treatment protocols. As expected, this pilot program, conducted in five districts, has shown a decrease in ACT consumption as RDT use is scaled up, resulting from a decrease in the number of false-positive malaria cases being treated with ACTs. Figure 5, below, documents the impact RDTs could have on ACT consumption as malaria diagnosis becomes more standardized and routine.

Figure 5. Results from PMI-supported RDT distribution in five seasonal epidemic-prone districts, from January 2011 through March 2012

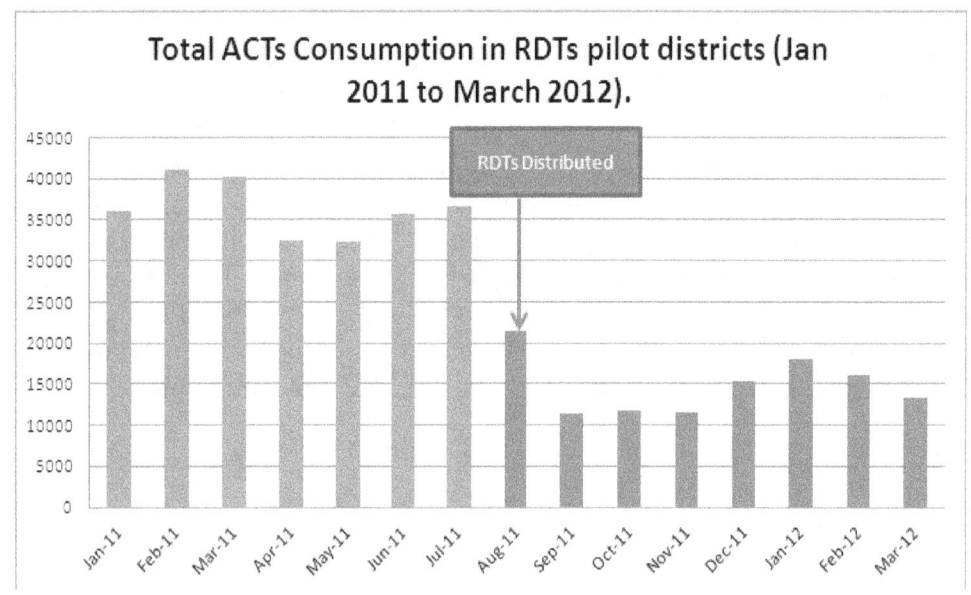

RDT Gap Analysis
Procuring sufficient RDTs to support the nation-wide roll-out of RDTs will be a challenge. Based on the DOMC's gap analysis, Kenya is expected to need 14.4 million RDTs in 2014. The Global Fund and PMI will work together to procure sufficient RDTs to fill the expected needs as calculated by the DOMC. Nonetheless, accounting for all donor contributions, the estimated

RDT gap through September 2014 is estimated to be 600,000, likely necessitating continued prioritization of RDT distribution to specific geographic regions and health centers.

As the DOMC strengthens malaria diagnosis at community and health facility levels, it is putting in place both a laboratory diagnostics quality assurance/quality control (QA/QC) program and a national malaria reference laboratory to coordinate laboratory-based parasitological testing at national and sub-national levels. The national malaria reference laboratory is a key component of a functional and transparent QA/QC program for both microscopy and RDTs. The reference laboratory will support all malaria intervention areas, including case management and malaria in pregnancy, vector control, epidemic preparedness and response, and surveillance, monitoring, evaluation and operational research. Support for the national malaria reference laboratory currently comes from the GOK and other malaria stakeholders.

The QA/QC system will work across the healthcare spectrum from the community to national levels when fully operational and is supported by PMI. The QA/QC system is being implemented at the district and health facility levels in Nyanza and Western provinces; these provinces have the highest prevalence of malaria in Kenya and are currently reliant on microscopy for diagnosis. The QA/QC system is in the development phase for the community (Level 1) and health dispensary (Level 2) levels. The QA officers at the district and health facility levels will be responsible for on-the-job training, capacity building, supportive supervision and adherence to diagnostic guidelines for RDT use at the community, dispensary and health facility levels. Because the QA/QC system relies on trained QA officers at the district and health facility levels, the current limited functionality of the national reference laboratory does negatively impact the system.

Progress to Date

PMI support for malaria diagnosis in Kenya is in line with DOMC priorities, which until recently have focused on increasing the availability of microscopes and the quality of microscopy at health facilities. In support of this, PMI procured 200 microscopes in 2010, and distributed a total of 175 of these in the Rift Valley, Nyanza, Western, Eastern, North Eastern, and Coast Provinces, with the remaining 25 going to the national reference laboratory. To further improve the quality of laboratory diagnosis of malaria, PMI is currently working with the DOMC, WHO and Office of the Chief Medical Technologist to implement a QA/QC system for the laboratory diagnosis of malaria in accordance with the WHO/CDC Laboratory Quality Management System.

A major component of the QA/QC system is the provision of supportive supervision and on-the-job training of health facility laboratory and clinical staff. A total of 80 laboratory technicians were trained in 2011, as well as 40 QA officers. These officers, some of whom are drawn from the pool trained by PMI in 2008, were trained using the WHO/CDC Laboratory Quality Management System Training Toolkit, WHO Malaria Microscopy Quality Assurance Manual, DOMC Laboratory Audit Checklist, and DOMC tools for RDT training. The QA officers were trained to undertake supervisory visits to assess staff capabilities, provide on-site remedial action, conduct internal and external quality assurance of malaria smear preparation and reading, and ensure correct usage of RDTs and ensure quality control of reagents and equipment.

A formal, centrally-supported QA/QC system is not currently operational in Kenya; strengthening this system will be a focus of PMI over the next two years with FY 2012 and FY 2013 funding. A plan for supervisory visits has been supported by PMI through an implementing partner at the provincial and district levels. The plan initially proposes supervisory visits only at facilities with laboratories; however, facilities without laboratories will receive additional training on the use of RDTs and supervision as a part of the nationwide RDT roll out.

Because the DOMC has not had sufficient RDTs in stock to conduct one nationwide distribution, PMI continued to support a targeted RDT roll-out in seasonal, epidemic-prone areas. As part of this support, PMI distributed 547,800 RDTs in 2011 to public health facilities. Of these, 110,600 were distributed to selected facilities in epidemic-prone districts, and 437,200 RDTs were distributed to all level 2-3 facilities (which include dispensaries, health centers and maternity/nursing homes) as part of the RDT pilot (results described above) in five selected districts in all four epidemiologic zones. As detailed in Table 7 above, both PMI and the Global Fund will continue to procure RDTs to support the goal of nationwide coverage, commensurate with the expected decrease in antimalarial need associated with an increase in the percent of fever cases tested.

In conjunction with the RDT roll-out, PMI also supported the training and supervision of laboratory and clinical staff in the correct use of RDTs, and worked with the DOMC to monitor the RDT roll-out process and gain experience needed to guide interventions aimed at improving health worker adherence to RDT results. PMI has also supported the DOMC by reviewing national laboratory policy guidelines and producing and disseminating appropriate job aids and standard operating procedures for both microscopy and RDTs.

Proposed PMI Activities with FY 2013 Funding: *($2,462,400)*

PMI will support the following malaria diagnostic activities:

1. *Procurement of RDTs:* In support of DOMC's RDT scale-up plan, procure and distribute up to 2 million RDTs to dispensaries and health centers in malaria endemic areas, as needed, to fill expected gaps. This will be done in coordination with other partner contributions. *($1,500,000)*

2. *Implementation support for RDT roll-out:* Provide funding for training, supportive supervision and monitoring of implementation of the RDT nationwide roll-out plan, including implementation of the QA/QC system, to ensure adherence to the DOMC policy guidelines for treatment and laboratory diagnostics. PMI will work with the DOMC and implementing partners to provide technical assistance and program implementation from the community to district and provincial levels to ensure a functional and robust laboratory diagnostics system for malaria. *($500,000)*

3. *Strengthen operations of the national reference laboratory:* Support and strengthen the operational capacity of the national reference laboratory via technical assistance and supplies/ consumables for the following national laboratory activities: *($150,000)*
   a. Proficiency testing of staff at national and peripheral levels
   b. Cross-checking of malaria blood films from health facilities by technical experts
   c. Training on and development of validation slide sets
   d. Consumables (e.g., slides, stains, supplies) to produce validation slide sets for 40 facilities quarterly
   e. Operationalization of the laboratory system to receive reports, slides, and results from peripheral levels and to generate and distribute results and reports to the peripheral levels

4. *Capacity building and supportive supervision within the established QA/QC system:* Strengthen and expand capacity for malaria laboratory diagnostics through training of QA officers at the district level, training and supportive supervision of laboratory and clinical staff by QA officers and supportive supervision of QA officers by technical experts, within the QA/QC system. The activities include initial and refresher training for QA officers, supportive supervisory visits to dispensaries and health facilities by QA officers to ensure adherence to laboratory guidelines and technical supervision of QA officers. *($300,000)*

5. *Technical assistance:* Support one CDC TDY to provide technical assistance for malaria laboratory diagnostics. CDC support will be focused on providing technical assistance for operationalization of the national laboratory and ensuring the implementing partner and DOMC develop a solid time line with a schedule for deliverables / milestones. *($12,400)*

Malaria Treatment and Pharmaceutical Management

Background

Kenya began dispensing artemether-lumefantrine (AL) as its first-line treatment for uncomplicated malaria in 2006. Aside from emphasizing the adoption of a diagnosis-based malaria treatment policy, the third edition of the National Guidelines for Diagnosis, Treatment, and Prevention of Malaria in Kenya adopted intravenous (IV) artesunate as the first-line treatment for severe malaria. Commensurate with this new policy will be the need for procurement and distribution of artesunate injections, updated trainings on the treatment of severe malaria, and quality of care for management of severe malaria.

Ensuring and maintaining access to proper antimalarial treatment remains a priority for the country. National stockouts, due primarily to slow procurement and delivery processes, have made ensuring an uninterrupted supply of AL to public health facilities a challenge over the past several years. As a result, the DOMC has prioritized efforts to accurately quantify stocks of AL and other antimalarial drugs, and implementation of evidence-based planning and appropriate distribution of AL stocks among facilities, good inventory management to avoid wastage of drugs through leakage and expiry, supervision/monitoring of availability of antimalarials, and information sharing through a logistics management information system.

PMI has supported antimalarial drug-quality monitoring at five sentinel sites since 2009; the activity is implemented by the National Quality Control Laboratory, Pharmacy and Poisons Board. With ongoing drug-quality monitoring, the National Quality Control Laboratory has strengthened surveillance and removed antimalarials of poor quality from the market. With funding from GOK, DFID and Global Funds (Round 4), the Pharmacy and Poisons Board has also developed pharmacovigilance guidelines and reporting tools and has performed sensitization of health workers; as a consequence, voluntary reporting of adverse drug reactions to antimalarials is being monitored by the Pharmacy and Poisons Board. In order to monitor the efficacy of current antimalarials, the DOMC has established sites to undertake *in vivo* drug efficacy monitoring to test the sensitivity of AL and examine the efficacy of new ACTs such as dihydroartemisinin-piperaquine (DHA-PPQ).

Due to the high percentage of persons who seek malaria treatment in private pharmacies and clinics, scaling up appropriate malaria treatment in the private sector and at the community level was a priority of the DOMC. In June 2010, the DOMC began implementing the Affordable Medicine Facility (AMFm), which was a two-year pilot program designed to expand access to affordable ACTs through public, private, and non-governmental organization supply chains by providing ACTs at a unit cost of US$0.05. The pilot program, which distributes ACTs to five registered private sector suppliers, will end in December 2012. Additional funding for program continuance is unlikely. With the end of the AMFm subsidy, the DOMC does not have alternate plans for scaling up appropriate malaria case management in the private sector in the 2009–2017 National Malaria Strategy.

Although the proportion of children with fever in Kenya who received prompt treatment with an ACT, as measured in the MIS, improved from 4% in 2007 to 11% in 2010, there is substantial room for improvement. The DOMC has begun to implement community case management of malaria (CCM) in Western and Nyanza Provinces by integrating it within the country's Community Strategy. Using Global Fund Round 10 funds, the DOMC is undertaking CCM preparatory activities in 2012, including procurement of ACTs and holding of community education meetings to increase awareness, compliance and provision of prompt treatment. By the end of 2012, it is expected that the development of CCM guidelines will be completed and up to 2,000 CHWs will be trained to provide health services at the community level.

Progress to Date

Pharmaceutical Management
To date, substantial progress has been made in the area of pharmaceutical management in Kenya with PMI support. PMI has helped maintain ACT stock levels to complement the Global Fund ACT procurements and to strengthen the supply chain to ensure an uninterrupted supply of ACTs to all public health facilities. PMI has procured large quantities of AL both on a planned and emergency basis, which has alleviated stockouts at the national level; however additional challenges remain. Public health facilities continued to experience stockouts during the past year, which highlighted the weak in-country logistic and supply chain systems. By the end of 2012,

PMI will have procured a total of over 25 million treatments of AL and distributed over 20 million to nearly 5,000 health facilities nationwide since 2008, and will continue to remain committed to ensuring that AL stockouts in Kenya do not occur. In addition to providing emergency stocks of AL, PMI worked with the DOMC, KEMSA and the Global Fund Principal Recipient to develop a supplier performance monitoring indicator to be included in future contracts.

PMI support for pharmaceutical management, including assistance with ACT quantification and distribution, supply chain strengthening, drug quality monitoring and case management supervision, has focused on health facilities, but has also helped in the DOMC's planned roll-out of CCM to Western and Nyanza Provinces.

Another major accomplishment is the implementation of the malaria commodity logistics management information system (LMIS), which monitors the availability of antimalarials and their respective consumption rates. Rolled out with PMI support in 2008, in response to a Global Fund requirement, LMIS is now operational in all districts in Kenya. PMI continues to sponsor monthly drug supply management sub-committee meetings to plan and monitor the stock situation for antimalarials.

Careful analysis of the LMIS stock and consumption data coupled with epidemiologic data has led to AL distribution being rationed throughout the country: the DOMC and the Kenya Medical Supplies Agency (KEMSA), the parastatal entity charged with the procurement, warehousing and distribution of public health commodities, have limited AL distribution in areas of low prevalence while increasing the availability and heightening the monitoring of ACT consumption in high prevalence areas. These efforts have more accurately matched the availability of AL to demand at the facility level, particularly in highly endemic areas.

PMI also supports semi-annual end-use verification facility surveys which assess the availability of malaria commodities at the end-user level, as well as provided a snapshot of how malaria was being diagnosed and treated at a sample of health facilities. In order for the end-use surveys to accurately guide the detection and correction of issues surrounding programmatic implementation, the DOMC requested that it be merged with a quality of care survey conducted by the Kenya Medical Research Institute (KEMRI)/Wellcome Trust. The coordination of DOMC, Wellcome Trust and PMI on this effort has turned the previously pilot-scale quality of care survey into a nationally representative survey, thus allowing the DOMC to use the findings to make improvements to case management. PMI has contributed to this effort by providing: technical assistance for the protocol development, with particular focus on the drug management component; support to train research assistants on drug management component data collection; logistical and financial support for data management; support for supervision of field work by the DOMC; and support for report writing, printing and dissemination.

After coping with chronic periodic national stockouts since 2007, Figure 6a below, shows that Kenya has not experienced a national stockout for over a year, which is a significant accomplishment for the GoK.

Figure 6a: Monthly Trend of ACT Stocks at the Central Level in Kenya, January 2011 – July 2012 (blue bar – total months of ACTs available)

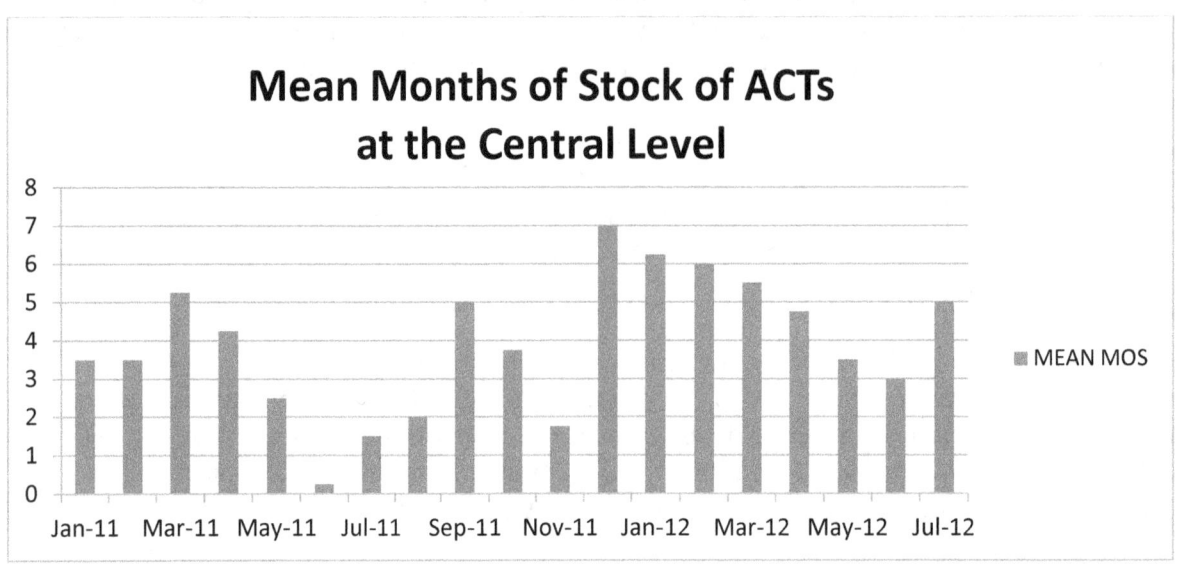

While facility stock levels still need improvement, over the same period of time that national stockouts were averted, sampled facilities have been able to maintain an average of 60% stock of all AL packs, and over 80% had at least one AL pack available. While encouraging, the DOMC and PMI recognizes that this is not good enough. PMI and the DOMC are working to eliminate stockouts at the district and facility levels, which is a top priority activity. Consequently, PMI is supporting KEMSA as the parastatal refines its distribution system to include a hybrid push-pull supply chain that incorporates more accurate quantification calculations from the facilities and districts. Additionally, PMI will support partners to work at the district level to improve quantification calculations to ensure timely orders of AL are sent to KEMSA. As part of this support, PMI will monitor the progress in reducing facility-level stockouts and functionality of the hybrid push-pull supply chain, by collecting routine data, in part with the following indicators:

- Percentage of facilities with all AL packs
- Percentage of facilities with at least one AL pack
- Percentage of facilities with SP
- Percentage of facilities with RDTs
- Percentage of facilities with injectable quinine
- Percentage of facilities with stockouts during the last 3 months
- Average length of stockouts
- Average time from beginning of facility stockout to district notification
- Average time from district notification to delivery of commodities

PMI will work with the DOMC to use these data, in combination with existing quality of care and end use verification surveys, to strengthen the performance of the malaria commodity supply chain.

Figure 6b: Monthly Trend of Stockouts of Non-Expired AL in Kenyan Health Facilities, January 2011 – July 2012 (blue bar – any AL stock; red bar – all AL packs)

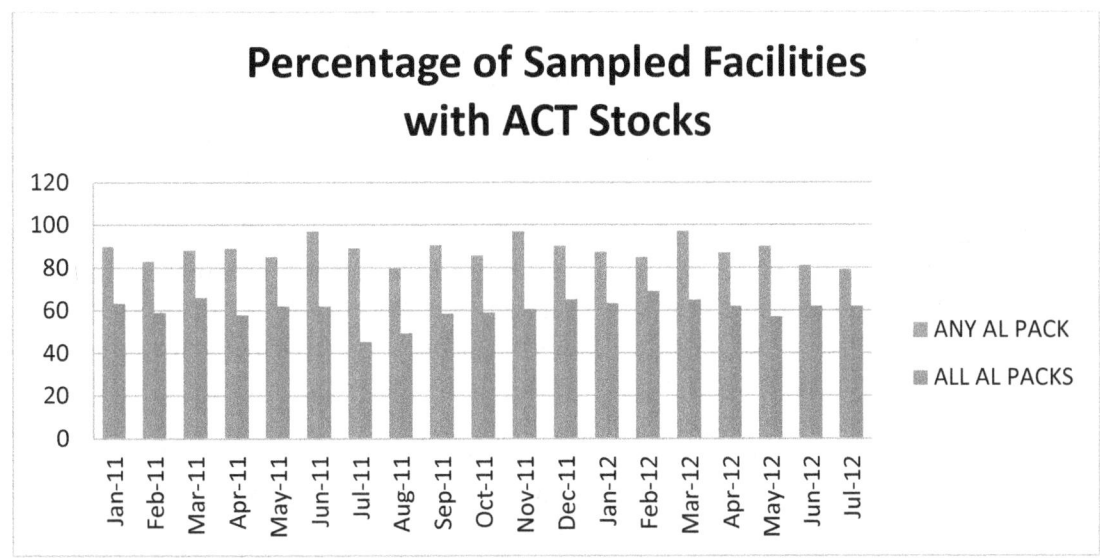

PMI continues to support an annual national quantification exercise to ensure that the AL requirements are being properly forecasted. DOMC quantification exercises estimated the country ACT needs through September 2014. While Table 7, below, confirms that the Global Fund Round 10 is scheduled to cover 100% of the anticipated ACT needs for the public sector facilities, this analysis does not include the buffer stock considered essential to ensure that national stockouts do not occur when stock management and drug procurement schedules are delayed. Further complicating the quantification calculations is that the Global Fund Round 10 Phase 1 grant funds reserved for AL procurements were negotiated based on the AMFm price of $0.05 per treatment, even for procurements scheduled to take place after December 2012 (when AMFm is scheduled to end). Without a clear picture of what the AMFm subsidy program will look like in January 2013, at the time of writing this MOP the DOMC remains uncertain exactly how much of the AL needs will be funded in the coming year. PMI continues to work closely with the DOMC to monitor the national AL stock needs and strives to fill commodity gaps to the greatest extent possible.

Table 7. Projected ACT needs and sources of funding for October 2012-September 2014

	October 2012-September 2013	October 2013-September 2014
Projected Need	16,700,000	13,900,000
Sources of Funding		
Global Fund	15,600,00	13,900,000
PMI	6,000,000	5,200,000
Projected Gap	**4,900,000**	**5,200,000**[A]
A. PMI ACTs will help fill the supply pipeline and ensure the availability of a 6 month buffer stock to alleviate potential stockouts due to delays in delivery of Global Fund-funded ACTs.		

PMI has supported antimalarial drug quality monitoring using Minilab® testing at five sentinel sites since 2009; the activity is implemented by the National Quality Control Laboratory, Pharmacy and Poisons Board. This activity allows Kenya to routinely provide evidence-based data on antimalarial quality and present data to policy makers for appropriate action and enforcement of medicine quality. In 2010, PMI supported the first round of drug quality monitoring using Minilab® testing, which revealed that 45 antimalarials were not registered, and 74 of the purchased products were expired. Further testing at the National Quality Control Laboratory revealed that seven antimalarial medicines failed quality control testing. The second round of Minilab® testing in 2011 showed the progress made to date; 22 antimalarials were not registered and 60 samples had expired. The results from these rounds allowed the Pharmacy and Poison Board to take effective corrective action against five companies and distributers that were unlawfully selling non-registered medicines. The Pharmacy and Poisons Board also issued a national recall and had the expired antimalarials withdrawn from the shelves. One manufacturer was closed down for selling unregistered and poor quality medicines.

In addition, PMI has conducted *in-vivo* drug efficacy testing in two selected sites in Western Kenya, and will continue to support drug efficacy monitoring. This activity evaluated the efficacy of the first- and second-line ACTs, AL and DHA-PPQ using standard WHO protocols, of determining cure rates on days 14 and 28 in children aged 6–59 months with uncomplicated *P. falciparum* malaria. Results confirmed that both AL and DHA-PPQ were equally efficacious, that there was no decay in sensitivity to AL over time, and both drugs were tolerable in children.

Training and Supervision
Training and supervision for malaria treatment management is being implemented through the new APHIA Plus Zone 1 bilateral, which provides integrated health facility services to all of Western and Nyanza provinces. This partnering allows PMI and the DOMC to take advantage of the significant PEPFAR resources used to build the foundation of the intervention; malaria-specific support is provided through the project to the hundreds of health facilities in the targeted areas. The APHIA Plus Zone 1 project was awarded later than expected, and therefore, results are not yet available for review by PMI. PMI will track this program closely to ensure that the supervision and training of health care providers progresses on time in order to ensure that the goals and objectives are met. It is anticipated that by the end of 2012, the project will have accomplished the following: finalized training materials for health facilities and community units, trained 500 health care workers on improved malaria in pregnancy services, trained over 74 district malaria coordinators as clinical mentors, established over 150 community units, provided supportive supervision (in coordination with district health management teams) in 10 districts. The work plan for the coming implementation year is being developed now; PMI and the DOMC anticipate the program to be operating at full capacity in 2013.

Proposed PMI Activities with FY 2013 Funding: *($6,825,000)*

PMI will undertake the following activities in support of malaria treatment:

1. *AL procurement*: Procure and distribute ~4.8 million AL treatments; if PMI is requested to fund new parenteral malaria drugs (i.e., injectable artesunate) by the DOMC, the number of ACT treatments procured and distributed will be reduced accordingly.

Funding for additional supply gaps, as needed, in the public sector through September 2014. *($5,200,000)*

2. *TA for supply chain management at national level and in-country drug distribution:* As the national supplier of medicines, including AL to the public sector health facilities in Kenya, PMI will support KEMSA to strengthen supply chain management, warehousing, financial management, and information systems. Support strengthening the system to a functional pull system, where KEMSA fills orders in a timely manner, based on complete reporting/documentation from the facilities. *($250,000)*

3. *TA for supply chain management at the district level:* Support to target lower levels of the antimalarial supply chain from district to facility level in the highly endemic districts. Key activities will include heightened monitoring of AL, SP and RDT availability, improving LMIS reporting rates, technical and financial support to the DOMC, Division of Pharmacy and district pharmacists to ensure effective quantification of drug and diagnostics needs, procurement, distribution and supervision of stock monitoring, on-the-job training and collection of antimalarial drug consumption data. *($575,000)*

4. *Strengthen drug quality monitoring and surveillance*: Strengthen antimalarial drug quality monitoring through the provision of technical, strategic and operational support to the Pharmacy and Poisons Board and DOMC. Support improved quality assurance of antimalarials and strengthening of pharmacovigilance. *($200,000)*

5. *Case management supervision*: Support the DOMC to strengthen malaria supervision and on-the-job training for case management in conjunction with the DHMTs. Activities will include promotion of prevention and treatment activities. *($600,000)*

6. *Technical assistance*: Support one visit from USAID to provide technical assistance for case management/drug procurement. *(Core funded)*

EPIDEMIC SURVEILLANCE AND RESPONSE

Background

Of the 16 epidemic-prone areas in Kenya (currently divided into 39 districts under the new organizational structure), three are in Nyanza Province, eleven are in Rift Valley Province and two are in Western Province. Four other seasonal transmission districts in the North Eastern Province also experience epidemics, usually associated with heavy rains and flooding. The total population of these districts is 6.5 million. Historically, Kenya relied primarily on case management for the control of epidemics, but over the last several years, the DOMC has been implementing preventive measures in these districts with the help of various partners.

Indoor residual spraying in the 16 epidemic-prone areas was started in 2006, supported through the Global Fund Round 4 grant. In 2008 and 2009, PMI supported IRS in two of these areas.

These two areas and the 14 other epidemic-prone areas in the DOMC IRS program were sprayed for the last time in 2010 as the DOMC refocused the IRS program on endemic districts. In place of IRS, an integrated disease surveillance and focalized epidemic response plan, combined with enhanced malaria surveillance, was implemented in 2010 after the withdrawal of IRS. In the malaria surveillance and response system, health centers submit data to districts on a weekly basis, and districts then transmit the data to provincial and national level by text message. Data is reviewed at the district level and case counts above preset thresholds are investigated by the district health officer. The district officer works with the Division of Disease Surveillance and Response (DDSR) and DOMC to validate the data, and in the event that there is a pocket of increased cases, the DOMC works with KEMSA/district health facilities to treat cases. Though there have been many investigations to date, progress still needs to be made to ensure a completely functional system: better communication of results between districts and the DOMC can improve, as can the DOMC's ability to respond to outbreaks in a standardized and effective matter.

Progress to Date

Maintaining a functional surveillance system that is able to detect unexpected increases in malaria cases is important to mitigating the extent of outbreaks in epidemic-prone areas. For this reason PMI will continue to support the epidemic surveillance and response system in epidemic-prone districts in Kenya. As outlined in the MOP text, this system has demonstrated the ability to collect quality data at the facility level, to calculate baselines upon which to identify epidemics, and the ability to transmit these data to the district level. The system has, however, thus far, failed to consistently transmit these data to the provincial and national levels. Both the successes and failures of this system were demonstrated in a recent outbreak in northeastern Kenya. Data collected at the facility level and transmitted to the district level aided in the targeted distribution of RDTs and ACTs; however, the DOMC encountered significant delays in obtaining these data from the DDSR when trying to analyze the effectiveness of their response.

Proposed PMI activities with FY 2013 Funding: *($200,000)*

PMI is using current funds to evaluate the system to identify the strengths and weaknesses, and the steps needed to be taken in order for the system to be fully functional. FY 2012 and FY 2013 funds will be used to address the weaknesses identified in the evaluation and ensure the implementation of corrective measures to strengthen the system. Because this evaluation has yet to occur, the specifics of the proposed activities are not yet known. Nonetheless, activities are likely to fall within the following areas:

1. *Implementation of surveillance, epidemic preparedness and response:* Implementation of the Epidemic Preparedness and Response plan, including improving malaria surveillance, updating and refining the national epidemic response plan, supporting the mapping of epidemic-prone areas, identification and training of health care workers in health facilities on epidemic preparedness and responses and generally enhance their capacity on malaria surveillance. (*This activity is budgeted under the M&E section*)

2. *Establishing epidemic preparedness stockpile:* In addition to maximizing ITN ownership and use in epidemic-prone districts through support of routine and mass ITN distribution described in the ITN section, PMI will support the procurement of supplies for epidemic response stockpiles in the epidemic-prone districts, including RDTs for diagnostics and ACTs and severe malaria medicines for large-scale treatment, if needed. Supplies will be held centrally and the supplies not used for epidemic response will be recycled through routine distribution channels to avoid expiry. *($200,000)*

BEHAVIOR CHANGE COMMUNICATION

Background

The NMS (2009-2017) aims to ensure that by 2014, 80% of the population in malaria-endemic regions has knowledge on the prevention and treatment of malaria. However, evidence from the 2010 National Malaria Indicator Survey demonstrated a low uptake of the treatment options albeit high knowledge level among respondents. In the survey, over 75% of household respondents were confident about hanging nets and agreed that children under 5 years of age should sleep under ITNs; however, only 42% of children under 5 years of age had slept under ITNs the previous night. In regard to treatment seeking behavior, over 90% of mothers of children under 5 years of age agreed that it was important to seek treatment promptly; IPTp2 uptake increased from 14% to 25%, however, only 11% of children received treatment within the stipulated period.

The DOMC has a national communication strategy developed in 2010 to guide and inform message development for malaria control interventions. Findings from studies carried out in the past by the ministry and other stakeholders in malaria control contributed to the development of the current strategy. The current communication strategy aims for social transformation by focusing on three key components: advocacy, communication and social mobilization. The strategy further segments audiences with corresponding key messages on each intervention. Previous studies have informed the selection of communication channels for each of the audiences based on the venue, content, frequency and timing of messages. The MoPHS also developed an Essential Malaria Action Guide for Kenyan Families in 2012, which outlines key messages and essential actions for each intervention area to ensure that all partners and stakeholders involved in malaria control are disseminating the same messages. The Essential Malaria Action Guide was developed in accordance with the Rollback Malaria Partnership's Strategic Framework for Malaria Communication at the Country Level, 2012–2017.

Progress to Date

PMI continues to support activities geared towards promoting the use of available malaria control tools by the most at-risk groups. In the last year, PMI supported a communication campaign in the aftermath of the 2011 mass ITN distribution effort to ensure that the over 7.6 million nets distributed during the campaign were actually being used by the recipients. PMI also supports the development of targeted messages to promote the use of nets among pregnant women and children under one year. In 2012, PMI supported activities in 15 of the 43 districts in the malaria endemic regions of Western, Nyanza and Coast Provinces. PMI funded support to local community-based organizations in these 15 districts to carry out different communication and promotional activities that address key messages on ITN use, prompt and appropriate treatment for malaria and ensuring that pregnant women have early ANC attendance to ensure the full dose of IPTp. Overall, in the past year, PMI has reached over 350,000 people in the 15 districts.

At the national level, PMI provided technical support in planning and in the development of a preparedness plan for an anticipated malaria outbreak in North Rift and North Eastern Kenya. In addition, PMI also supported the development and production of IEC materials that informed and alerted communities in the regions about the malaria epidemic expected during the short rains in September to December. Health worker job aids and guidelines on the use of intravenous artesunate for severe malaria treatment were produced. During the same period radio messages were also placed during prime time in different ethnic languages. In addition, PMI supported the production of District Malaria Control Coordinators Manuals for the programmatic management of malaria at the district level.

During this first year of support to the Peace Corps initiative, Stomping Out Malaria, PMI funds facilitated targeted assistance to two volunteers in Nyanza and Western Province to help them continue promoting behavior change and increasing acceptance of key malaria prevention and treatment interventions. However one of the Peace Corps volunteers left the country for further studies. The remaining volunteer worked with the provincial Malaria coordinator and an implementing partner to facilitate education through listening sessions. These are sessions held with small groups (approximately 9–12 participants) of community members to enhance interaction and reflections on topical issues related to malaria control within the community. The participants in the sessions are led by a facilitator. The facilitator introduces the topic for discussion and each of the participants is given an opportunity to contribute to the topic discussion while the others listen and critique after the presentations. Finally, all the participants reach a consensus and agree on individual and community actions to take in regards to malaria control activities.
PMI will continue support for the operational costs for up to three volunteers through the end of 2012.

Proposed PMI Activities with FY 2013 Funding: *($1,030,000)*

With FY 2013 funding, PMI will continue to support IEC/BCC activities. Specific activities include:

1. *Targeted community-based IEC/BCC in endemic and epidemic-prone districts:* Expand community-based IEC/BCC to cover more districts from the current 15 to 20 districts by increasing outreach to priority populations, especially pregnant women and children under five years, through different strategies and channels of communication. Messages and modes of dissemination will depend on the venue and target population. Interpersonal communication will be used during home visits by CHWs, while *barazas* will be held in villages and during public gatherings where messages are delivered

through public address systems. During these gatherings, skits and dramas will be used to deliver messages on malaria control in a more engaging manner in order to:

- Increase ITN ownership and promote correct and consistent use of ITNs;
- Promote early and regular ANC attendance by pregnant women to increase the proportion of women using IPTp; and
- Increase early and appropriate health-seeking behavior and prompt management of fever. *($700,000)*

2. *National IEC/BCC efforts:* With the DOMC issuing its new malaria control strategy, and revising its policies and guidelines regarding IPTp and RDTs (among others), it requires assistance with national-level IEC efforts. PMI will support national-level IEC message development and dissemination on key malaria control interventions related to the new policies and guidelines (i.e., MIP, case management, diagnosis, IRS, etc.). The DOMC will work with partners to roll out the new messaging on the use of IPTp for malaria in pregnancy as indicated by the new epidemiological changes of malaria endemicity. PMI will also support the DOMC to roll out RDTs in all parts of the country initially beginning in low transmission zones and moving to the rest of the country. In order to inform, enhance, and increase the acceptance of RDTs among health workers and communities, PMI will support the development and production of IEC materials with information on RDTs. PMI will also work with other partners and coordinate donors to undertake advocacy-related activities, including regular review meetings with donors to monitor and guide their progress in malaria control interventions. This will help to ensure that malaria control remains a national priority. *($300,000)*

3. *PMI-Peace Corps collaboration*: Under the PMI-Peace Corps Initiative, Peace Corps has recruited three Malaria Support Volunteers who will work under the guidance of PMI country advisors and closely with the host government and other stakeholders to support malaria control activities at the district level where they will work with the District Malaria Control Coordinators (DMCC). The Peace Corps will provide technical support to community-based groups (CBOs) working in malaria control interventions at the district level. PMI will support these three Peace Corps volunteers with resources to carry out BCC activities in any of the intervention areas namely - IRS, ITNs, MIP and case management, as well as in cross-cutting areas of capacity building and surveillance, monitoring, evaluation and operations research as identified by the respective District Health Management Teams (DHMTs). *($30,000)*

4. *Technical assistance*: Support one visit from USAID to provide technical assistance for the implementation of the IRC/BCC program. *(Core funded)*

INTEGRATION WITH OTHER GLOBAL HEALTH INITIATIVE PROGRAMS

Kenya is a GHI plus country and has developed a strategy that embraces the key tenets of the initiative. GHI Kenya seeks to establish a robust whole-of-government, multi-layer communication strategy, reflecting all fundamental principles of the President's initiative. This will benefit the full complement of the USG health portfolio in Kenya. GHI Kenya builds upon the existing interagency management platform. Building on a solid interagency governance system, GHI Kenya makes appropriate modifications to the structure already functioning in country. US Peace Corps, Department of Defense, CDC, USAID and President's Emergency Plan for AIDS Relief (PEPFAR) have implemented and reported on a large program base for several years. This tight, multi-tiered governance structure allows for full participation across agencies, at all levels, and across technical areas – resulting in well-conceived programs that are responsive to country needs.

In Kenya, GHI adds new dimensions to the existing disease-focused structure. GHI Kenya embraces a strong management base and expands into broader public health areas relevant to the GHI Strategy. GHI Kenya emphasizes the development of programs that leverage unique capacities of each of the agencies, utilizing existing activities and platforms to create efficient and functional cross-agency synergies. Over time, this model will mature into expanded inter-agency work to achieve GHI objectives and targets under the learning agenda.

PMI in Kenya has been working closely with the Walter Reed Army Institute of Research. Walter Reed has received funding from PMI/Kenya in previous years to purchase and distribute microscopes and to provide training on microscopy for malaria. Walter Reed has also assisted in finalizing the DOMC's National Diagnostics Guidelines and is currently working to develop and implement an external quality assurance program for malaria microscopy in support of DOMC and PMI malaria control activities.

PMI in Kenya is in the process of expanding its collaboration with Peace Corps. Under a renewed effort to "Stomp Malaria Out of Africa", Peace Corps-recruited Malaria Support Volunteers will work under the guidance of PMI country advisors and closely with the host government and other stakeholders to support malaria control activities within the existing national malaria control plan.

CAPACITY BUILDING AND HEALTH SYSTEMS STRENGTHENING

Background

The DOMC is responsible for planning, organizing, and coordinating all malaria control activities in the country. It is also responsible for developing training and implementation guidelines for all the intervention areas through the different technical working groups. The DOMC has 24 staff members at the national level, four physicians, one PhD entomologist, four public health officers, three clinical officers, two pharmacists, three nurses, one health records officer and various other support staff. These officers are assigned as focal point persons to the following interventions: vector control, surveillance, monitoring and evaluation and operational research, advocacy communication and social mobilization, epidemic preparedness and response, malaria in pregnancy, case management and diagnostics, and program management. In the spirit of decentralization of malaria control operations, malaria focal persons at the district and soon-to-be county level have been designated and trained in malaria management (including planning, budgeting, decision making, supervision, and M&E). The malaria focal points are staff within the MOPHS who take on additional responsibilities to support malaria control activities. With these new responsibilities, the district and county malaria focal points require training to bring them up to speed with the latest malaria control strategies, policies, and guidelines that are being rolled out.

The focal points at the DOMC are required to conduct supervisory field visits together with the district and provincial focal points to assess how interventions are being implemented. However these visits tend to occur in an ad hoc manner due to inadequate planning, and do not achieve the intended results of ensuring that services are delivered as expected and corrective measures are taken where needed.

With the new constitution and the division of the country into 47 new counties (from the current eight provinces and 158 districts), devolution of governance, management, coordination of services, and the oversight of health service delivery continue to evolve. New challenges in coordination, service delivery and staff capacities are expected. In order to address these challenges the DOMC needs to ensure that staff in these new county structures are adequately trained to plan and manage the implementation of malaria control activities based on the needs of the district/county or province.

It is expected that human resources development and organizational management skills will be needed to successfully operate under the new county structures and processes where the malaria focal points will likely take on more direct responsibilities for disease control operations than occurs under the current system. Increasing skills in this area will ensure that malaria control teams are able to face the new challenging circumstances under which they will be working. They will get training in problem solving approaches, leadership skills, managing change, communication, etc.

However, a lack of sufficient funds and logistical issues may continue to challenge the DOMC's ability to adequately supervise and support staff through this transition.

The DOMC technical working groups (TWGs) serve as a way of engaging key partners and overseeing implementation of programs. Currently there are six TWGs, including the: 1) Drug Policy Technical Working Group, 2) IEC Working Group, 3) MIP Working Group, 4) Vector Control Working Group, 5) Surveillance, Monitoring, Evaluation and Operational Research Working Group, and 6) Case Management Working Group. The groups are comprised of all key partners working in a specific technical area, with the DOMC acting as the secretariat. The groups meet either quarterly or on an ad hoc basis to address emerging issues. The TWGs report regularly to the Malaria Interagency Coordinating Committee. Continued support to the TWGs is important, especially for those TWGs that are less active.

Progress to Date

DOMC Capacity Building
PMI has continued to support the DOMC to fulfill its responsibilities in conjunction with other partners. PMI's DOMC capacity building efforts work towards a stronger GOK and a more sustainable malaria control program. Previous PMI support to the DOMC has included training and supervision of health workers to ensure that they are in compliance with the new treatment guidelines. Building on work in previous years in M&E, PMI currently supports the DOMC to

ensure timely collection of quality health information through the Malaria Information Acquisition System and the national HMIS, and has supported two DOMC officers to attend international trainings in M&E and Health System Management. Additionally, PMI has supported training for 54 DOMC officers in two malaria M&E workshops on data analysis and M&E report writing.

Through support to the TWGs, PMI strengthens policy dialogue and supports the development of appropriate tools, interventions, guidelines, strategies and policies that promote effective integrated management of malaria, pharmaceutical system strengthening and program monitoring.

Contributions to Health System Strengthening
PMI strengthens the overall health system by improving governance in the pharmaceutical sector, strengthening pharmaceutical management systems, expanding access to essential medicines, and improving service delivery. Over the past year, PMI supported the implementation of the malaria commodity LMIS, facilitated emergency AL distribution, and improved drug quality monitoring. PMI is working with the DOMC and Office of the Chief Medical Technologist to implement a QA/QC system for malaria diagnostics.

To build human resource capacity and improve service delivery, PMI has continued to support the training of health workers at the facility and community levels.

Proposed PMI Activities with FY 2013 Funding: *($550,000)*

PMI will use FY 2013 funds to continue to improve the DOMC's technical capacity, help it fulfill its leadership role, and to ensure the strengthening of the technical working groups. (Some health systems strengthening activities are incorporated into activities funded in the different intervention areas). Specifically, PMI will fund the following:

1. *PMI direct technical support to DOMC:* Provide technical support by USAID and CDC PMI Advisors to the DOMC. These Advisors will spend a portion of their work week with the DOMC and will have a workstation within the DOMC offices to effectively integrate into the national team. *(no additional cost)*

2. *Support for DOMC (Total of $250,000):* Three main activities -

   a. *DOMC capacity building:* Improve the DOMC's technical capacity with regard to implementation and supervision. PMI's funding will enable the DOMC focal point persons to supervise and track malaria prevention and control activities carried out in priority districts. Support for these supervision activities will be undertaken in collaboration with other Ministry of Health officers, to create synergy and strengthen the overall malaria program management. *($200,000)*

   b. *Attendance of DOMC staff at technical consultative meetings:* Assist DOMC focal point persons to keep abreast with the latest developments and advances in the field of malaria control by attending key technical meetings (such as the East

Africa Regional Network or inter-country meetings organized to discuss monitoring and evaluation). Attendees will be expected to make presentations and share key technical updates with other DOMC members. *($25,000)*

    c. *Support the DOMC Technical Working Groups:* PMI in collaboration with other development partners will lead efforts to ensure the TWGs are strengthened, functioning effectively and efficiently, and holding regular meetings to establish and identify key topical issues in malaria control that need to be addressed in order to enhance the overall achievement of planned goals for the program. *($25,000)*

3. *Decentralization to the new county system:* PMI will support the DOMC's efforts to operationalize malaria control efforts within the new 47-county administrative system to ensure that the delivery and coordination of malaria prevention and control activities and services in the new counties are not disrupted. Strengthened malaria coordinators at the county level will ensure the management and operationalization of new county-level programs. They will help align the DOMC with the new decentralization and the DOMC's role in the new process, establish their role in the new context and define the new role of the counties by becoming active players and engaged in the discussion. They will be expected to provide critical links within the new decentralized system between the DOMC and the sub-county operations to ensure that programs continue to operate and function well. It is expected that by 2014, PMI will be supporting the county structures directly through existing partnerships to ensure support at the county level, beyond technical assistance. *($300,000)*

4. *Health systems strengthening in supply chain management, health worker training, laboratory strengthening, and district-level supportive supervision:* Described in the case management section.

COMMUNICATION AND COORDINATION WITH OTHER PARTNERS

There are a number of very active partners in malaria control in Kenya, including research institutions, non-governmental organizations, WHO, DfID, the private sector and development partners that work closely with the DOMC and each other through both formal and informal structures. PMI is an integral partner with the DOMC and actively participates in all technical and other partner-related activities.

A malaria subgroup under the Malaria Interagency Coordination Committee is convened by the head of the DOMC on behalf of the Director of Public Health. It includes the Ministry of Health, non-governmental organizations, faith-based organizations, the private sector and development partners. This group meets quarterly with additional interim meetings occurring as needed. There are also several technical working groups led by the DOMC around particular issues. These include the Drug Policy Technical Working Group, which was convened to help implement Kenya's drug policy change; a formal IEC working group which comprises representatives from various departments of the MOPHS and stakeholders to assist in the implementation of the IEC strategy and plan; a MIP working group; an integrated Vector Control working group; a

Surveillance, Monitoring, Evaluation and Operational Research working group; and a Case Management working group.

MONITORING & EVALUATION

Background

DOMC framework for monitoring and evaluation
Effective monitoring and evaluation of the malaria control program has been prioritized in the NMS 2009-2017 as an essential function of DOMC program management. The goal is to assess progress made towards achieving set program objectives and targets as laid out in Objective Four "To strengthen surveillance, monitoring and evaluation systems so that key malaria indicators are routinely monitored and evaluated in all malarious districts by 2011 through capacity strengthening for malaria surveillance, routine monitoring and operational research." The DOMC has a Surveillance, Monitoring, Evaluation and Operational Research unit which is mandated to coordinate the generation of information on the progress of malaria intervention implementation, the evaluation of programs, support supervision, data auditing for quality, data dissemination and use. The unit is equipped with the requisite hardware and software to enable data compilation, analysis and storage in an M&E database.

Since 2009, the DOMC and its stakeholders have been using one comprehensive national M&E framework (DOMC M&E plan, 2009-2017) to enable transparent and objective management of information on the national malaria control activities. Kenya has a large number of stakeholders with the interest and capacity to conduct effective surveillance, monitoring, evaluation and operational research. Key M&E stakeholders (drawn from government, universities, research institutions, private sector, non-government organizations and donor agencies) are organized into a surveillance, monitoring, evaluation and operations research technical working group to collectively provide guidance on the DOMC's M&E activities. Overall, malaria data flow within the M&E framework is from the community to the district, provincial and national levels, as well as to DOMC partners. It is anticipated that with the new devolved government structure, data flow will move from the sub-county to county to national level. The M&E plan articulates the program objectives by intervention area; lists key indicators; highlights required data and data sources; reviews the institutional arrangements for gathering, analyzing, and reporting data, and for investing in capacity building; and states the ways in which M&E findings will be fed back into decision making. The costed M&E work plan is used for M&E advocacy, communications and resource mobilization.

Data Sources and Reporting Systems
The types and sources of data for DOMC M&E indicators include:

1. Routine disease and service reporting and national surveillance from the HMIS, LMIS, Laboratory Information Management System (LIMS), the Integrated Disease Surveillance and Response (IDSR) system, and district, provincial and national administrative systems. In 2013, with the devolution of government, the information systems will be revised to include data from the county level.

2. Routine sentinel surveillance information from five sites monitoring antimalarial drug quality and two sites monitoring antimalarial drug efficacy. With decreasing malaria risk in the country, sentinel health facilities established in 2000 to collect data representative of the four different epidemiologic zones, are no longer routinely used by the DOMC/KEMRI/Wellcome Trust to collect retrospective data on implementation and health impact of malaria control interventions.

3. Routine demographic sentinel information from Kenya's Demographic Surveillance System (DSS) sites in Kisumu (population of 135,000, managed by KEMRI/CDC) and Kilifi (population of 220,000, managed by KEMRI/Wellcome Trust). In the absence of functional national vital registration systems, these sites monitor birth and death rates, mortality and morbidity rates, socioeconomic indicators, and conduct verbal autopsies to ascribe probable causes to all deaths.

4. Non-routine DOMC activity information on ITN, IRS, IPTp and case management activities, generated and transmitted vertically following activity implementation by the DOMC and implementing partners supported with Global Fund, DfID/WHO and PMI funds.

5. Non-routine survey information gathered from health facilities, schools, communities and households [e.g., DHS, MIS, Multiple Indicator Cluster Survey, Service Provision Assessment (SPA), national census].

6. Non-routine information from ongoing malaria-related research and special studies including operational research.

The DOMC, donors and partners use these data sources to monitor program implementation and assess program impact. Table 8 summarizes the available data sources and assessments in Kenya since 2005 and planned activities.

Table 8. Timeline of Data Collection Activities in Kenya

Data Source	Year									
	2005	2006	2007	2008	2009	2010	2011	2012	2013	2014
DHS				X					X	
MICS				X[i]						
MIS			X[i]			X				X
SPA						X				
RIA								X		
MPR					X					X
EUV/QoC					X	X	X	X	X	X
HMIS[ii]	X	X	X	X	X	X	X	X	X	X
IDSR[iii]		X	X	X	X	X	X	X	X	X

[i]The 2007 MIS and 2008 MICS were subnational.
[ii]DHIS started in 2010 to provide improved district-level facility data collection.
[iii]IDSR began scaling up in 2006.

While the DOMC uses routine information to track changes in program performance over time, impact and outcome measurements of the program and population-based coverage are estimated through facility and household surveys and routine surveillance (HMIS, DSS).

Notable strengths of the Kenyan malaria M&E system include the organizational structure of the M&E unit; M&E partnerships; and the presence of a comprehensive M&E system and costed M&E plan. The main weakness, as reported by Data Quality Assessments conducted in 2010 by the Global Fund and Kenya's Ministry of Public Health and Sanitation, is the delay in data made available through the HMIS. An audit by the Regional Inspector General in 2012 also indicated a lack of information and clarity on tracking malaria commodities at the lower levels (e.g., district health facilities).

The DOMC implements most malaria M&E activities through funding from the Global Fund and PMI, with additional support from DfID. Available funding is targeted towards achieving:

1. Improved functioning of M&E unit resources (existing technical capacity, available hardware and software capability, and satisfactory information dissemination);
2. Coordination of malaria M&E within the country;
3. Improved data flow from all data sources;
4. Data quality assurance; and
5. Using data for decision making.

Progress to Date

PMI has supported the measurement of the outcome and impact indicators listed below by providing support for the malaria component of the 2008-09 DHS and the 2010 MIS:

Indicators:
- All-cause under-five mortality
- Proportion of households with at least one ITN
- Proportion of children under five years old who slept under an ITN the previous night
- Proportion of pregnant women who slept under an ITN the previous night
- Proportion of women who received two or more doses of SP during their last pregnancy in the last two years, at least one of which was received during an ANC visit
- Proportion of children under five years old with fever in the last two weeks who received treatment with ACTs within 24 hours of onset of fever

PMI has previously supported reporting of complementary data on malaria-related morbidity and mortality in the KEMRI/CDC DSS. PMI has also been supporting *in vivo* antimalarial drug efficacy monitoring. In addition, PMI is providing support to the DOMC's acquisition and storing of routine data through the Malaria Information Acquisition System (MIAS) and for strengthening the quality and timeliness of data from various data sources.

In addition, PMI has provided technical assistance to support malaria M&E coordination, improved data flow, data quality assurance and use of data for decision making. PMI has done this by building DOMC/M&E capacity at the national level. As capacity is built, the DOMC/M&E staff are able to strengthen their national DOMC counterparts as well as provincial- and district-level M&E staff with support from the Global Fund and PMI.

Within the last 12 months, PMI has:

- Supported M&E capacity building in the DOMC by providing technical assistance for the DOMC's M&E and governance structures including the M&E TWG. Support has also been provided to the Operations Research TWG and Malaria Inter-Agency Coordinating Committee. Additionally, PMI funded two DOMC focal points to attend malaria M&E and Health Systems Management trainings.

- Further capacity building was achieved by facilitating two five-day M&E training workshops on the fundamental concepts and practical approaches to malaria M&E. These were held in Nairobi for 54 Government of Kenya officers drawn from the district, provincial and national level. Through PMI support, the local implementing partner conducted a follow-up survey of the workshop trainees to assess knowledge retention and data use activities. The results indicated that there was a marked improvement of knowledge of malaria and M&E concepts; pre-test scores averaged at 59% versus 76% in the first post-test. A second post-test was conducted six months after M&E training. Over half of the officers trained completed the second post-test, and overall scores on the second post-test were higher than those during the pre-test. The majority of respondents reported finding the training useful/helpful for carrying out their work in the six months since the course and had applied the knowledge and skills they learned in the training to their current work. A total of 83% of respondents reported that they have shared their data with stakeholders and/or partners in the past six months.

- Assisted with the strengthening of the malaria surveillance systems by supporting the development of a national malaria surveillance strategy, finalizing an assessment of the gaps in indicator collection from the main data sources (HMIS and IDSR) and developing a plan of action for implementation of the DOMC's updated comprehensive surveillance activities. The development of these comprehensive surveillance system activities are being planned based on WHO guidance. Kenya's changing epidemiology and its vision of being malaria-free have emphasized the need for robust routine surveillance data for use in guiding intervention planning and emergency response as the country transitions from high transmission to low transmission to pre-elimination. PMI is supporting the strengthening of the routine surveillance system along with Global Fund and other partners.

- Designed a District Malaria Control Coordinator (DMCC) malaria surveillance tool comparing passive and mixed (i.e., passive plus active) models that was piloted in six districts and conducted a sensitization workshop on the use of the tool, interpretation of core surveillance graphs and electronic data upload. The passive data collection model relied on the DHIS data being compiled by the DMCC, whereas the mixed model utilized the DHIS data but also involved the DMCC going to the health facilities. The next steps over the coming 12 months are the development of a report documenting the lessons learned, results and recommendations from the pilot, including recommendations on which data collection model to use (i.e., passive or mixed). Following the release of the findings and recommendations, a plan will be developed through a consensus-building workshop and then rolled out to all malarious districts.

- Organized the logistics and facilitated the first Kenya National Malaria Forum: Moving from Evidence to Action, held October 10-11, 2011 in Nairobi. As the DOMC unit continues to monitor progress, it has determined the need to harness the efforts of individuals, institutions and organizations at all levels of the health care system involved in the generation and use of malaria data to better inform its control strategies and policies. The DOMC used the forum to review the latest malaria research evidence to inform the country's malaria programs and strategies. The planning process was deemed successful in generating content for the forum based on an integrated participatory process including a review of the data needs and policy gaps by the DOMC focal point persons and broader malaria stakeholders in Kenya. Presenters for these topic areas were then selected through a call for abstracts and targeted invitations, including representatives from the Rwanda and Senegal NMCPs to share examples from other endemic countries. The forum was also deemed a success for fostering a discussion among the 135 participants about data needs for the various malaria topic areas and recommending operations research to address these.

- A Data Quality Audit for USAID/Kenya PMI was completed in July 2012 to assess the Data quality Management System (DMS) in Kenya and second, to establish the precision, validity and integrity of data reported to USAID/Kenya. Four key monitoring indicators were reviewed: 1.) Number of Artemisinin-based combination therapy (ACTs) purchased and distributed using USG funds, 2.) Number of insecticide treated nets (ITNs) purchased with USG funds, 3.) Number of insecticide treated nets (ITNs) distributed or sold with USG funds, and 4.) Number of rapid diagnostic kits (RDTs) purchased and distributed through USG support. The auditors visited nine GOK health facilities, a KEMSA warehouse and PSI offices. The audit report cited a key strength being that the electronic systems used by KEMSA and PSI are "…accurate and trust-worthy. There are many built in QC cross-checks built into these systems." Vulnerabilities were also identified with recommendations to improve the quality of data and reporting on PMI indicators. PMI and the USAID Kenya Mission will follow-up on the recommendations in the DQA report to improve the quality of the data being reported to the mission and PMI. Improving collection of the four indicators that were the target of the DQA assessment is also likely to improve the reporting and quality of additional indicators (e.g. commodity procurement and distribution indicators) being used to monitor PMI activities in Kenya as they are collected through similar reporting mechanisms.

- In 2010 and 2011, PMI provided financial and technical support to module design, field work, data analysis and report writing for the 2010 MIS. Recently PMI supported technical participation in the MIS dissemination workshop held in the Lake endemic region.

Proposed PMI Activities with FY 2013 Funding: *($2,375,000)*

With FY 2013 funding, PMI will continue to support malaria M&E within the framework of the National Malaria M&E Plan (2009-2017) as follows:

1. *M&E implementation*: Continue support for implementation of the national M&E plan by providing technical assistance to increase the capacity of existing DOMC M&E staff and to ensure that data is used for program improvements. Specific activities are listed below. *($500,000)*
   - Provide support to the strengthening of routine surveillance systems including incorporation of relevant malaria indicators, such as IPTp uptake, into the HMIS and DDSR systems in order to heighten surveillance in different epidemiologic settings. The DOMC uses the DDSR information to prevent and respond to epidemics. Specifically, FY 2013 funding will help the DOMC ensure the generation of quality data; encourage data use by supporting performance review meetings, supervision and decision making; and undertake monitoring and evaluation (including feedback, supervision and system improvements). The DOMC has requested continued PMI support for malaria surveillance across endemic areas in addition to epidemic surveillance.
   - Support the improvement of the quality of data collected through routine systems by supporting the standardization of forms, improving supervision, conducting data checks, and participating in annual Data Quality Audits. This will ensure that data collected through the routine system is of sufficient quality to be utilized for malaria surveillance and epidemic detection.
   - Support the DOMC in reviewing and identifying the reasons for declining use of the MIAS. This will include addressing identified deficiencies so that the MIAS is a functional system that allows data collection, storage, and use in a way that meets the DOMC's needs.
   - Provide technical assistance to the DOMC in planning the 2014 MIS.
   - Support the DOMC in the analysis and presentation of data for quarterly reports, briefs for policy makers and journalists, and for updates on the DOMC website. Support the DOMC in the generation of its Annual Malaria Report.
   - Organize an annual malaria review meeting for stakeholders.

2. *Malaria Indicator Survey*: Support the collection of malaria control intervention outcome and morbidity indicator data through the 2014 MIS. Based on a schedule of conducting an MIS survey every three years and a DHS survey every five years, both surveys are due in 2013. In order to avoid two surveys in the same year, the DOMC postponed the next MIS until 2014. The 2014 MIS will allow the DOMC to evaluate intervention coverage, anemia and parasitemia. PMI will only support the collection of parasitemia data in children 6-59 months of age. Parasitemia data from 2014 will be compared against parasitemia levels in the 2007 and 2010 MIS surveys to track national progress towards reducing the malaria burden and to monitor transitions from high burden to low burden to pre-elimination. It is anticipated that the MIS will cost roughly $1.8 million and DfID and Global Fund have both committed to fund portions of the 2014 MIS. Due to concerns

about the availability of funds during the transition from Phase 1 to Phase 2 of the Global Fund Round 10 grant, PMI will designate funds for the 2014 MIS, based on a funding gap analysis by the DOMC, to ensure the MIS proceeds according to the DOMC's schedule (fieldwork tentatively beginning in July 2014). If Global Fund Round 10 Phase 2 funds become available, PMI will contribute to fill any remaining funding gap and will reprogram the remainder of these funds. *($1,000,000)*

3. *Strengthen the health information system at the district level*: The Health Management Information Systems has recently launched the DHIS that gathers routine data at the health facility level and in the near future at the community unit level. The DHIS will be integrated with the LMIS allowing for the coordination of health service and commodity statistics. The DHIS is a sector-wide information system, of which malaria is one component. The DOMC is heavily reliant on the HMIS since it is not a vertical program in that it uses the health systems that are already in place to collect routine data. The DHIS has the potential to be extremely useful to the DOMC, and the opportunity to ensure malaria is a centerpoint of the DHIS will need to be harnessed. The real time access to surveillance data will also aid the DOMC in better responding to potential epidemics. PMI is providing support to the $32.8 million project over five years, funded primarily through PEPFAR. PMI and the DOMC will leverage this funding by PEPFAR and take advantage of the ongoing investment in improving HMIS to gather additional malaria data at the district level. This activity will benefit the DOMC and assist the DOMC in collecting timely malaria data at the district and community level. There are three clear deliverables that PMI's funding will go towards: 1) support establishment of a national IT infrastructure to support the rollout of a national integrated health and management information system (service statistics, HR, finance, commodities etc. that GOK would develop today and in the near future), 2) support development of a learning and knowledge management system that produces information products and services that match information needs of all programs in the health sector including malaria and, 3) build capacity of the HIS division to adequately implement the functions of the division. This project will support the DOMC not just in availing data through DHIS but in ensuring that DOMC uses this data for program improvement. Funding from PMI funding will support the DOMC in ensuring malaria indicators are included in the DHIS to improve data collection and informed decision making for malaria programs. *($200,000)*

4. *Monitoring of interventions*: Support M&E activities for specific intervention areas which are fully described under the relevant technical sections: *($550,000)*

   a. Monitor stock status and avert stockouts through the use of the End Use Verification tool. The activity will be done semiannually as part of the DOMC's Quality of Care survey so as to allow the DOMC to design holistic recommendations to improve case management. Approximately 170 of the 5713 health facilities will be randomly sampled each time, for a total of 340 health facilities sampled per year. The facilities will include dispensaries, health centers and hospitals owned by the GOK, faith-based organizations and NGOs across seven of the eight provinces (excluding Nairobi). Global Fund funding will also support this activity. *($100,000)*

b. Conduct epidemiologic surveillance in endemic IRS districts and comparison districts to monitor human malaria infections to inform the DOMC's IRS intervention strategy. This will include health facility-based disease burden monitoring designed to monitor malaria burden over time and to provide the DOMC with data that will guide the scale-down of IRS in the wake of universal ITN coverage. In areas where IRS is withdrawn, this surveillance will enable detection of a potential resurgence in malaria cases. *($175,000, see the full activity description in the IRS section)*

c. Conduct continuous monitoring and evaluation of MIP activities in targeted endemic districts, specifically monitoring the effect of implementation of the revised IPTp policy. This will include specific monitoring of the supportive supervision activity such as the quality of supervision provided and health provider perceptions and practice. At the end of the intervention, an evaluation will be undertaken to determine the uptake of IPTp2 among pregnant women. *($75,000, see the full activity description in the IPTp section)*

d. Support epidemiologic surveillance in highland and seasonal transmission districts for epidemic detection. This activity will include implementation of the Epidemic Preparedness and Response plan, with a focus on improving malaria surveillance. *($200,000, see the full activity description in the Epidemic Surveillance and Response section)*

5. *Field Epidemiology and Laboratory Training Program:* Train two FELTP trainees for a two-year secondment, upon graduation, to the DOMC. As there is very low attrition in the MOPHS among the graduates of this program, PMI anticipates that this investment will increase the long-term capacity within the DOMC to be able to carry out appropriate program planning, implementation and monitoring and evaluation. The DOMC requested PMI funding for training of additional staff to support the various M&E and surveillance activities. PMI will now support two new FELTP trainees each year, as opposed to alternate years as has been done previously. These additional trainees are likely to play an important role as devolution of the government proceeds and there is a need for additional staff trained in malaria M&E at the county level. PMI will work with the head of the FELTP program in Kenya to give priority to Ministry of Health staff already working on malaria for these FELTP trainee positions. The budget for each trainee includes tuition, stipend, laptop, materials, training, travel, and conferences for the two-year program. *($100,000)*

6. *Technical Assistance:* Support two CDC TDYs to provide technical assistance for M&E activities. *($25,000)*

7. *Technical Assistance*: Support one USAID TDY to provide technical assistance for M&E activities. *(Core funded)*

STAFFING AND ADMINISTRATION

Two health professionals have been hired as Resident Advisors to oversee PMI in Kenya, one representing CDC and one representing USAID. In addition, a third health professional, a full-time FSN staff member, has been hired to join the PMI team. All PMI staff members are part of a single interagency team led by the USAID Mission Director. The PMI team shares responsibility for development and implementation of PMI strategies and work plans, coordination with national authorities, managing collaborating agencies and supervising day-to-day activities.

The three PMI professional staff work together to oversee all technical and administrative aspects of PMI in Kenya, including finalizing details of the project design, implementing malaria prevention and treatment activities, monitoring and evaluation of outcomes and impact, and reporting of results. The USAID staff members report to the Director of the Office of Population and Health at the USAID/Kenya Mission. The CDC Resident Advisor is supervised by CDC, both technically and administratively. All technical activities are undertaken in close coordination with the Ministry of Health/DOMC and other national and international partners, including WHO, DfID, Global Fund, World Bank and the private sector.

Locally-hired staff to support PMI activities either in Ministries or in USAID will be approved by the USAID Mission Director. Because of the need to adhere to specific country policies and USAID accounting regulations, any transfer of PMI funds directly to Ministries or host governments will need to be approved by the USAID Mission Director and Controller.

Proposed PMI Activities with FY 2013 Funding: *($1,115,200)*

- *In-country PMI staff salaries, benefits, travel and other PMI administrative costs*: Continued support for two PMI (CDC and USAID) and one FSN (USAID) staff members to oversee activities supported by PMI in Kenya. Additionally, these funds will support pooled USAID Kenya Mission staff and mission-wide assistance from which PMI benefits. *($1,115,200)*

Table 1: Kenya Year 6 (FY 2013) Budget Breakdown by Partner

Partner Organization	Geographic Area	Activity Description	Activity Budget	Partner Subtotals
Afya Info	Nationwide	Strengthen the Health Information System and the collection of information at the district and community level	$200,000	$200,000
APHIA Plus HCM	Endemic/Epidemic districts	Logistic support to routine and mass campaign ITN distribution	$1,800,000	$3,380,000
	Selected priority endemic districts	Support implementation of a continuous ITN distribution system	$300,000	
	targeted endemic districts in Nyanza, Western and Coast	Integrated community-based IEC/BCC	$700,000	
	Nationwide	National IEC promotion	$300,000	
		Peace Corps support	$30,000	
		Support to DOMC	$250,000	
APHIA plus "Zone 1"	Zone 1 (includes 2 provinces -Nyanza and Western)	Strengthen malaria supervision for case management	$600,000	$600,000
CDC IAA (with sub-grant to KEMRI)	Endemic Districts	Entomological monitoring of IRS effectiveness in sprayed districts	$180,000	$579,800
	5 Endemic Districts	Epidemiologic surveillance in endemic IRS districts	$175,000	
	priority endemic districts in Nyanza, Western and Coast	Support continuous MIP monitoring in endemic districts	$75,000	
CDC IAA (Atlanta)	Endemic Districts	CDC IRS TDY visit	$12,400	
	Nationwide	CDC Diagnostics TDY support	$12,400	
	Nationwide	CDC M&E TDY support	$25,000	
	Nationwide	Train 2 field epidemiology and laboratory training program epidemiologists	$100,000	

57

Implementer	Location	Activity	Amount	Total
DELIVER	Endemic/Epidemic districts	Procure ITNs for routine distribution and 2014 mass distribution campaign	$8,100,000	$15,000,000
	Nationwide	Procure RDTs	$1,500,000	
		Purchase AL and/or severe malaria medication	$5,200,000	
	targeted district(s)	Stockpile epidemic response equipment and supplies	$200,000	
HCSM	Nationwide	Provide support to the DOMC for implementation of RDTs	$500,000	$1,175,000
		TA for supply chain management at district level	$575,000	
		Support the end-use verification tool/Quality of Care Survey	$100,000	
HPP	Nationwide	Facilitate decentralization to new county system	$300,000	$300,000
IRS TO2	Endemic Districts	IRS implementation and management	$7,000,000	$7,000,000
MEASURE Evaluation	Nationwide	Support for implementation of the National M&E plan	$500,000	$500,000
MVDP (Walter Reed)	Nationwide	Strengthen the operations of the national reference laboratory	$150,000	$450,000
		Provide supportive supervision within the established QA/QC system for the national laboratory network	$300,000	
TBD	Nationwide	Strengthen antimalarial drug quality monitoring and surveillance	$200,000	$2,100,000
	priority endemic districts in Nyanza, Western and Coast	Support supervision of FANC/IPTp program	$450,000	
	Nationwide	TA for supply chain management at national level and in-country drug distribution	$250,000	
	Nationwide	Support for 2014 MIS	$1,000,000	
	Epidemic-prone/seasonal districts	Implementation of surveillance, epidemic preparedness and response	$200,000	
USAID/CDC	Nationwide	In-country administration and staffing	$1,115,200	$1,115,200

FY 2013 Budget Total $32,400,000

Table 2: Kenya Year 6 (FY 2013) Planned Obligations

Proposed Activity	Mechanism	FY 2013 Budget	FY 2013 Commodities	Geographic area	Description of Activity
Insecticide Treated Nets					
Procure ITNs for routine distribution and 2014 mass distribution campaign	DELIVER	$8,100,000	$8,100,000	Endemic/Epidemic districts	Fill the ITN gap for routine distribution and mass campaign by purchasing up to 1.8 million LLINs. Routine distribution: free-of-charge to pregnant women and children under one through the ANC and child welfare care clinics. Nets are estimated at $4.50 each.
Logistic support to routine and mass campaign ITN distribution	APHIA Plus HCM	$1,800,000	$0	Endemic/Epidemic districts	Provide logistical support, including transportation and storage of nets, for distribution of the 1.8 million ITNs within the national routine distribution system and mass distribution campaign.
Support implementation of a continuous ITN distribution system	APHIA Plus HCM	$300,000	$0	Selected priority endemic districts	Continue strengthening Kenya's continuous ITN distribution system to maintain high coverage levels achieved through mass distribution efforts. This activity will identify and close distribution gaps and promote cost effective tracking systems to ensure that populations living in targeted districts will be able to replace ITNs as they wear out, with the ultimate goal of ending the need for mass campaigns to keep ITN coverage at optimal levels.
USAID TDY visit	USAID	$0	$0	Nationwide	Support one visit from USAID to provide assistance in implementing the ITN program (Core Funded).
Subtotal		**$10,200,000**	**$8,100,000**		
Indoor Residual Spraying					
IRS implementation and management	IRS TO2	$7,000,000	$2,310,000	Endemic Districts	Support IRS in up to three endemic districts with a target of 85% coverage of targeted households in all districts, includes emergency focal spraying in epidemic districts (as needed), and TA to DOMC for spray operations.
Entomological monitoring of IRS effectiveness in sprayed districts	CDC IAA (with sub-grant to	$180,000	$0	Endemic Districts	Continue insecticide resistance monitoring in endemic districts targeted for spraying by PMI in western Kenya

Activity	Mechanism		Coverage		Description
	KEMRI				
CDC IRS TDY visit	CDC IAA (Atlanta)	$12,400	Endemic Districts	$0	Support one visit from CDC to provide assistance in implementing IRS activities.
Subtotal		**$7,192,400**		**$2,310,000**	
Malaria in Pregnancy					
Support supervision of FANC/IPTp program	TBD	$450,000	Priority endemic districts in Nyanza, Western, and Coast	$0	Supportive supervision to continue correct implementation of the simplified IPTp guidelines in facilities and at the community level for all targeted malaria endemic districts. This activity builds on the facility-based investments already undertaken and aims to strengthen demand for and provision of IPTp at ANC in all 55 targeted districts.
Subtotal		**$450,000**		**$0**	
Case Management					
Diagnostics					
Procure RDTs	DELIVER	$1,500,000	Nationwide	$1,500,000	In support of DOMC's RDT scale-up plan, procure and distribute 2 million of the required RDTs to dispensaries and health centers in targeted districts.
Provide support to the DOMC for implementation of RDTs	HCSM	$500,000	Nationwide	$0	Provide funding for DOMC to engage with the QA officers to ensure quality supportive supervision, support full roll-out of RDTs and monitor implementation, to ensure adherence to DOMC RDT policy guidelines throughout the country.
Strengthen the operations of the national reference laboratory	MVDP (Walter Reed)	$150,000	Nationwide	$150,000	Purchase consumables for NRL operations that will be scaled-up by 2013. Microscopy is being used to test samples coming into the NRL. Staff will need advanced training on microscopy and eventually training on PCR techniques. The supply chain/logistics support for transporting samples (logistics, methodologies, etc. maintenance of this activity) will need to be established. As the country rolls out RDTs, there is a need to ensure results of RDTs are reliable. NRL will ensure quality of this new diagnostic tool and validate results for providers.

Activity	Mechanism			Location	Description
Provide supportive supervision within the established QA/QC system for the national laboratory network	MVDP (Walter Reed)	$300,000	$0	Nationwide	Strengthen capacity for malaria diagnostics through supportive supervision of district level QA officers, within the QA/QC system. Includes: refresher training of QA officers, validate RDTs as they are rolled out, technical supervision of adherence of testing guidelines.
CDC Diagnostics TDY support	CDC IAA (Atlanta)	$12,400	$0	Nationwide	Support one CDC TDY to provide technical assistance for malaria diagnostics.
Treatment					
Purchase AL and/or severe malaria medication	DELIVER	$5,200,000	$5,200,000	Nationwide	Procure and distribute up to 4.8 million AL treatments and severe malaria drugs, as needed, to fill in supply gaps in the public sector through September 2014. Procure severe malaria drugs, (injectable artesunate), as needed.
TA for supply chain management at national level and in-country drug distribution	TBD	$250,000	$0	Nationwide	As the national supplier of medicines, including AL to the public sector health facilities in Kenya, PMI will support KEMSA to strengthen supply chain management, warehousing, financial management and information systems. Support strengthening the system to a functional pull system, where KEMSA fills orders in a timely manner, based on complete reporting/documentation from the facilities.
TA for supply chain management at district level	HCSM	$575,000	$0	Nationwide	Support to target lower levels of the antimalarial supply chain from district to facility-level in the highly endemic districts. Key activities will include heightened monitoring of AL, SP and RDT availability in the high endemic districts, improving LMIS reporting rates, technical and financial support to the DOMC, Division of Pharmacy and district pharmacists to ensure effective quantification of drug and diagnostic needs, procurement, distribution, and supervision of stock monitoring, on-the-job training, and collection of antimalarial drug and RDT consumption data.
Strengthen antimalarial drug quality monitoring and surveillance	TBD	$200,000	$0	Nationwide	Strengthen antimalarial drug quality monitoring through the provision of technical, strategic and operational support to the PPB and DOMC. Support improved quality assurance of antimalarials.

Activity	Description	Location	Amount	Amount	Implementer
Strengthen malaria supervision for case management	Support the DOMC to strengthen malaria supervision and on-the-job training for case management in conjunction with the DHMTs. Activities will include promotion of prevention and treatment activities.	Zone 1 (includes 2 provinces - Nyanza and Western)	$600,000	$0	APHIA plus "Zone 1"
USAID TDY visit	Support one USAID TDY to provide assistance for CM/Drug Procurement (Core Funded).	Nationwide	$0	$0	USAID
Subtotal			**$9,287,400**	**$6,850,000**	
Epidemic Surveillance and Response					
Stockpile epidemic response equipment and supplies	Support the procurement of supplies for epidemic response stockpiles in the targeted districts, including: IRS for focal spots, RDTs for diagnostics and ACTs and severe malaria medicines for large-scale treatment, if needed.	Targeted district(s)	$200,000	$200,000	DELIVER
Subtotal			**$200,000**	**$200,000**	
IEC/BCC					
Integrated community-based IEC/BCC	Expand community-based IEC/BCC efforts by increasing outreach to priority populations especially pregnant women and children under five years through different strategies and channels of communication. Messages and mode of dissemination will be dependent on the venue and target group. In hospitals, at the ANC clinics, interpersonal communication will be used as well as in homes during home visits by community health workers, while *Barazas* will be held in villages and during public gatherings where messages are delivered through public address systems.	Targeted endemic districts in Nyanza, Western and Coast	$700,000	$0	APHIA Plus HCM
National IEC promotion	Support national-level IEC message development and dissemination on key malaria control interventions on the new policies, and donor coordination, undertake advocacy-related activities, including regular review meetings with donors working in the malaria constituency to monitor and advise on their progress in malaria control interventions.	Nationwide	$300,000	$0	APHIA Plus HCM
Peace Corps support	Continue PC activities and support three malaria PCVs.	Nationwide	$30,000	$0	APHIA Plus

Activity	Partner	Cost	Location	Description
	HCM			
USAID TDY visit	USAID	$0	Nationwide	Support one USAID TDY visit to provide assistance for IEC/BCC Program (Core Funded).
Subtotal		**$1,030,000**		
Capacity Building and Health Systems Strengthening		**$0**		
Support to DOMC	APHIA Plus HCM	$250,000	Nationwide	Provision of technical assistance and capacity building to improve the DOMC's technical capacity to fulfill its role in support to implementation and supervision; ensure the technical working groups are strengthened and hold regular meetings.
Facilitate decentralization to new county system	HPP	$300,000	Nationwide	Strengthen malaria coordinators at the county level to ensure that they are able to manage county-level programs that are new and need to be operationalized. Help align the DOMC with the new decentralization and the DOMC's role in the new process, establish/define their role in the new context and define the new role of the counties. Become active players and engaged in the discussion. Expect that by 2014 we will be supporting the county structures. Working at the county level, resources need to move down to this level; not just TA, but actual support to the county levels.
Subtotal		**$550,000**		
Monitoring and Evaluation		**$0**		
Support for implementation of the National M&E plan	MEASURE Evaluation	$500,000	Nationwide	Continue support for implementation of the national M&E plan by providing technical assistance to increase the capacity of existing DOMC M&E staff and to ensure that data is used for program improvements. Support for technical assistance for malaria surveillance and improvement of the MIAS.
Support for 2014 MIS	TBD	$1,000,000	Nationwide	Support the 2014 Malaria Indicator Survey.

Activity	Implementer	Budget		Location	Description
Strengthen the Health Information System and the collection of information at the district and community level	Afya Info	$200,000	$0	Nationwide	Support HMIS's recently launched District Health Information System (DHIS) which gathers routine data at the health facility level and in the near future at the community unit level. The DHIS will be integrated with the LMIS. Ensure malaria information is captured through the DHIS.
Support the end-use verification tool/Quality of Care Survey	HCSM	$100,000	$0	Nationwide	Monitor quality of care for malaria case management and the LMIS to assess stockouts through the end-use verification tool.
Epidemiologic surveillance in endemic IRS districts	CDC IAA (with sub-grant to KEMRI)	$175,000	$0	5 Endemic Districts	Support epidemiological surveillance and monitoring in endemic IRS districts. The surveillance will include support for improved surveillance at select health facilities in the IRS districts in order to monitor prevalence changes over time and to provide the DOMC with data that will guide the IRS strategy in the wake of universal LLIN coverage, and detect any potential resurgence i n cases with IRS is withdrawn.
Support continuous MIP monitoring in endemic districts	CDC IAA (with sub-grant to KEMRI)	$75,000	$0	Priority endemic districts in Nyanza, Western and Coast	Support monitoring of MIP activities in targeted endemic districts, including specific monitoring of MIP interventions where new guidelines are disseminated with supportive supervision and enhanced community BCC activities.
Implementation of surveillance, epidemic preparedness and response	TBD	$200,000	$0	Epidemic-prone/seasonal districts	Implementation of the Epidemic Preparedness and Response plan, including improving malaria surveillance, updating and refining the national epidemic response plan, supporting the mapping of epidemic-prone areas, identification and training of health care workers in health facilities on epidemic preparedness and responses and generally enhance their capacity on malaria surveillance.
Train two field epidemiology and laboratory training program epidemiologists	CDC IAA (Atlanta)	$100,000	$0	Nationwide	Train two FELTP trainees for a two-year secondment, upon graduation to the DOMC to increase the long-term capacity within the DOMC to carry out appropriate program planning, implementation and monitoring and evaluation. The budget for each trainee includes tuition, stipend, laptop, materials, training, travel.

CDC M&E TDY support	CDC IAA (Atlanta)	$25,000	$0	Nationwide	Support two CDC TDYs to provide technical assistance for M&E activities.
USAID M&E TDY support	USAID	$0	$0	Nationwide	Support one USAID TDY to provide technical assistance for M&E activities. (Core Funded).
Subtotal		**$2,375,000**	**$0**		
Staffing and Administration					
In-country administration and staffing	USAID	$715,200	$0	Nationwide	USAID staffing and mission wide support efforts.
In-country administration and staffing	CDC IAA (Atlanta)	$400,000	$0	Nationwide	CDC Advisor staffing and support costs.
Subtotal		**$1,115,200**	**$0**		
GRAND TOTAL		**$32,400,000**	**$17,460,000**